GW00891257

Strategies managing the menopause

by **Dr Jean Coope** MD, FRCGP

General Practitioner, Macclesfield, Cheshire

PUBLISHING
INITIATIVES
BOOKS

Doral House • 2(b) Manor Road • Beckenham
Kent BR3 5LE

My thanks are due to Henry Burger, the Chairman of the World Health Organisation Scientific Group on the Menopause 1994, and Barbara Hulka who edited the report. The British Menopause Society has been helpful and my work as Editor of the *Journal of the BMS* has put me in touch with a variety of research workers, academics and 'ordinary' doctors. The Macclesfield Hospital Postgraduate Library and the Department of Medical Illustration at Wythenshawe Hospital Manchester have provided references and illustrations.

Finally, I would like to thank our knowledgeable and hard-working research secretary, Joyce Marsh, who put the manuscript together.

A NOTE ABOUT THE AUTHOR

Dr Coope started research into the menopause and hormone replacement therapy in 1974 and has pioneered the prevention of osteoporosis in general practice, offering screening and education to women in middle life.

She has written numerous articles and taken part in radio and television broadcasts. She was a member of the WHO Scientific Research Group on the Menopause and is the Editor of the *Journal of the British Menopause Society*.

First Published in Great Britain 1996
This edition reprinted 1997

ISBN 1 873839 37 5

Further copies of *Strategies for Managing the Menopause* may be obtained from Pi books, a division of Publishing Initiatives (Europe) Ltd. This publication reflects the view and experience of the author, and not necessarily those of Publishing Initiatives (Europe) Ltd.

Printed and bound in Great Britain by Prospect Litho Printers Ltd., Maidstone, Kent ME20 7AR.

It is a great pleasure and privilege for me to provide a foreword for this most useful and practical book. *Strategies for Managing the Menopause* will benefit all of us who are involved in prescribing for, counselling and managing women around and after the time of the menopause and those taking hormone replacement therapy (HRT). I believe that the benefits of HRT are now well established, not only for symptoms such as hot flushes, for which Jean Coope was the first to demonstrate the true effect of oestrogen by a properly controlled double-blind placebo cross-over trial, but also for the long-term benefits on the skeleton and cardiovascular system. However, in order to achieve the latter benefits, a woman must take HRT for several years and all the surveys on continuation rates have shown that very few achieve this. Women, their doctors and other medical advisers are often uncertain about the risk/benefit ratio, and also how to manage the side-effects of HRT and other problems with therapy which may affect compliance. Jean Coope has been at the forefront of menopause research for more than 20 years and her very successful menopause clinic achieves annual continuation rates of 84-92%, which are much higher than anyone else has reported. This book, therefore, gives us some of the secrets of how she achieves such results, and it is full of good, sensible, practical advice.

There are so many new HRT preparations being released that it is becoming very difficult for even the menopause experts to keep up to date with them all. However, this is less important, perhaps, than the principle of therapy and prescribing, and awareness of the ways in which adjustments can be made to relieve side-effects and problems. Throughout the book the emphasis is on counselling and giving correct and easily assimilated information, and on encouraging the woman to feel she is in control of the situation. This is important now when it is evident that women learn so much about the menopause and HRT from the mass media, and often this information is sensationalist, anecdotal, incorrect and sometimes anti-HRT. Recent publicity for vitamins and other dietary supplements, and the use of various foods containing progesterone-like substances, is presented in such a way that the public are led to believe that there is some scientific validity in these statements. In reality none of these alternative remedies has been subjected to controlled trials, and they may just be providing a placebo response.

Having the support of a book such as this will be a great help to all those who are trying to help women through the difficult problems of the menopause and post-menopausal years. I am quite certain, too, that our great mentor and the grandfather of modern HRT, the late Robert Greenblatt, would have advocated and enjoyed this book. He strongly believed that women should not have to accept a 'change of life' and in true scholarly fashion in one of his essays he wrote:

"A woman in the autumn of her life deserves an Indian summer rather than a winter of discontent."

I hope this book will help us all in the pursuit of this goal.

Dr David Sturdee MD FRCOG
Consultant Obstetrician and Gynaecologist, Solihull Hospital
Chairman of the British Menopause Society

BMC	bone mineral content
BMD	bone mineral density
CABG	coronary artery bypass graft
CES-D	Centre for Epidemiological Studies Depression Scale
CNS	central nervous system
COC	combined oral contraceptive
CSM	Committee on the Safety of Medicines
D&C	dilatation and curettage
DEXA	dual energy X-ray absorptiometry
DHEAS	dehydroepiandrosterone sulphate
ERT	estrogen replacement therapy
FMP	final menstrual period
FSH	follicle-stimulating hormone
Gn-RH	gonadotrophin-releasing hormone
HDL	high-density lipoprotein
HRT	hormone replacement therapy
IHD	ischaemic heart disease
IUD	intrauterine device
LDL	low-density lipoprotein
LH	luteinising hormone
LH-RH	luteinising hormone-releasing hormone
LMP	last menstrual period
MI	myocardial infarction
MPA	medroxyprogesterone acetate
MSSU	mid-stream specimen of urine
OPCS	Office of Population Censuses and Surveys
QCT	quantitative computed tomography
QoL	quality of life
RCT	randomised controlled trials
SD	standard deviation
SEM	standard error of the mean
SHBG	sex hormone-binding globulin
THBG	thyroid hormone-binding globulin
WHO	World Health Organisation

Evidence-based medicine is becoming fashionable nowadays and nowhere is it more important than in the field of managing the menopause. What is the menopause? Is it anything more than the cessation of periods? Are there any symptoms which are specific to that time of life and do they respond to hormone therapy? These questions have been answered by a series of population studies and clinical experiments during the past 20 years. The consensus seems to be that psychological symptoms, such as depression, are not related to the hormonal changes of the menopause but are triggered by pre-existing negative perceptions and social problems made worse by the youth-orientated culture in which we live. Middle-aged women are anxious as they approach what they perceive as a looming disaster, although afterwards they often comment that the menopause was a minor event in their busy lives.

Nevertheless, the years go on, bones become fragile and arteries are clogged. The post-menopausal woman is increasingly at risk from osteoporosis and heart disease, and there is a wealth of evidence to support the provision of HRT as a preventive treatment. In spite of this, doctors and patients are often reluctant to accept long-term therapy for healthy patients who may or may not develop symptoms in the future. We are on the horns of a dilemma. The value of long-term oestrogen in the prevention of cardiovascular disease and fractures is recognised yet there is considerable anxiety about side-effects, particularly the possible increased risk of breast cancer in older women.

A further problem is the tendency of women of higher social class and greater education to select themselves as HRT users. The poor and ignorant less often attend health promotion clinics, smoke more heavily and use less HRT than their better-off sisters. Observational studies, which compare users with controls, have this major confounding factor, particularly in the field of cardiovascular disease, that those most at risk are least likely to take oestrogen. The case for long-term HRT cannot be finally clinched without a large-scale randomised trial. One is already under way in the United States, under the auspices of the National Institutes for Health, and the Medical Research Council has organised a similar trial in the UK. Until we can allow for the effects of social class, income and education on women's health, doctors are working in the dark. We assume that oestrogen with or without progestogen is cardioprotective, but how large is its effect?

Older women are more likely to suffer from fractures or heart disease, but recent research suggests[1] that they may also have a higher risk of breast cancer on HRT. Weighing risks and benefits for the individual and providing expert counselling usually falls to the lot of the primary health-care team. This work is skilled and time-consuming, and is difficult to compress into an ordinary practice consultation. A new breed of practice nurse is growing up, trained in preventive care and able to undertake education and supervision of menopausal patients. They need the back-up of informed doctors and the whole primary care team can only be adequately served by critically reviewed evidence that is as up-to-date as possible. This book attempts to provide the scientific basis for advice and prescription for those who are working at the grass roots of medicine.

The rise and rise of medical research means that textbooks are quickly out of date: what was 'true' about the menopause at the time of writing will not necessarily be 'true' 10 years, or even one year, later. I can only ask the reader to accept the transient nature of medical science and to update the evidence where it has been proved fallible.

Reference

1. Colditz GA, Hankinson SE, Hunter DJ et al. The use of estrogens and progestins and the risk of breast cancer in post-menopausal women. N Engl J Med 1995; **332**: 1589-93.

CHAPTER **ONE**

The symptoms and how to manage them

What is meant by the word 'menopause'?

L iterally this means that a woman's periods have stopped. However, there is a great deal of confusion and in order to avoid ambiguity we are adopting the definitions used by the report of the World Health Organisation Scientific Group Meeting in 1994 (*in press at the time of writing*).

- Natural menopause: the permanent cessation of menstruation resulting from the loss of ovarian follicular activity. It is recognised to have occurred after 12 consecutive months of amenorrhoea, for which there is no other obvious cause, and can be known with certainty only in retrospect, a year after the final menstrual period (FMP).

  An adequate **biological** marker for the event does not exist.

- Perimenopause: includes the period immediately before the menopause, when endocrinological, biological and clinical features of approaching menopause commence, and the first years after menopause.

- Premenopause: should encompass the entire reproductive period up to the FMP.

- Post-menopause: dates from the FMP, whether induced or spontaneous.

- Induced menopause: includes removal or other iatrogenic ablation of both ovaries.

- Simple hysterectomy: with conservation of one or both ovaries defines a separate group in which ovarian function may persist for a variable period after surgery.

- Premature menopause: is defined as occurring at an age less than 2 SD below the median for the referred population. Because of lack of data, the age of 40 years is often used as an arbitrary cut-off point.

There are 470 million women in the world who are past the menopause; because we are living longer this figure is growing rapidly and will exceed 1.2 billion by the year 2030. Most of these women are poor and will be living in developing countries without access to sophisticated medical technology, yet the menopause is important to them. Although traditionally the menopause is associated with transient symptoms, such as hot flushes, these pale into insignificance compared with the post-menopausal problems of osteoporosis and heart disease which are both related to oestrogen deficiency. Although there are differences in incidence between different ethnic groups, there is a worldwide problem of osteoporosis and fractures in elderly women, which are becoming more frequent all over the world (*Figures 1.1 and 1.2*).

Figure 1.1 Patterns of hospital admission for fracture for women in the Trent Region of England 1989/90[1].

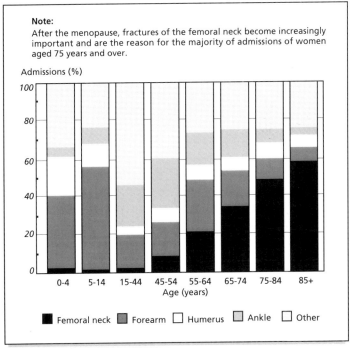

Note:
After the menopause, fractures of the femoral neck become increasingly important and are the reason for the majority of admissions of women aged 75 years and over.

Admissions (%)

Femoral neck   Forearm   Humerus   Ankle   Other

Reproduced with the permission of WHO from: Assessment of fracture risk and its application to screening for post-menopausal osteoporosis: Report of a WHO study group. Geneva, World Health Organization, 1994 [Technical Report Series, No 84].

3

Figure 1.2 Estimated number of fractures for men and women in different regions of the world in 1990, 2025, and 2050[2].

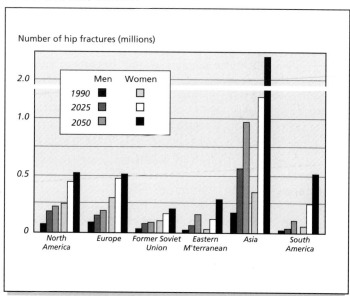

Reproduced with the permission of WHO from: *Assessment of fracture risk and its application to screening for post-menopausal osteoporosis: Report of a WHO study group. Geneva, World Health Organization, 1994* [Technical Report Series, No 84].

In the UK, there are more than 60,000 hip fractures and 90,000 wrist and vertebral fractures each year, mostly occurring in women over 50 years of age[3].

The leading cause of death in Western women is ischaemic heart disease and this accounts for nearly 30,000 deaths a year in this country, mostly before the age of 75. (*Office of Population Censuses and Surveys, 1992*)

The average age of death of British women is now over 80, so many occurring before 75 can be regarded as premature deaths. Both osteoporotic fractures and ischaemic heart disease are partly preventable. Reduction of circulating oestrogen increases women's vulnerability[4]; this can be improved by judicious use of HRT and other measures, such as stopping smoking, exercise and a healthy diet, which depend in turn on educating women. The overwhelming need and the cost-effectiveness of women's education is now recognised and was a major theme of the World Conference on Women in Beijing, September 1995.

Doctors need educating too. It is noteworthy that in 1991 a survey of over 1,000 general practitioners in the Medical Research Council general practice research framework found that only 9% of their female patients aged 50-64 were receiving HRT[5]. The menopause is a time when doctors and patients should take stock and decide whether they need to take long-term preventive measures against future illness and early death.

Other problems more closely related in time to the menopause include hot flushes, night sweats and insomnia, urinary symptoms and sexual difficulty due to vaginal atrophy. All these affect the quality of life, and all respond to oestrogen therapy.

What happens at the menopause?

Menstruation ceases and hormonal levels change (*Figure 1.3*).

Figure 1.3 Plasma levels of estradiol and testosterone in human females and males according to age[6].

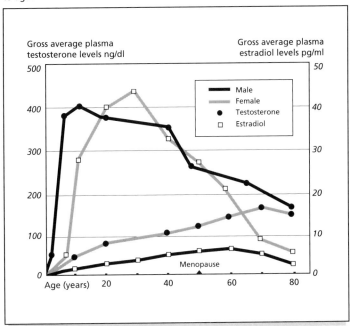

Reproduced with the permission of the author.

Endocrinology

The ovary secretes two types of hormone: the steroids, oestradiol and progesterone; and the peptides, inhibin and activin. Oestradiol and the peptides are produced by the granulosa cells of the ovarian follicle. Progesterone is secreted by the corpus luteum which is formed from the follicle after ovulation. Peak levels are dependent on the occurrence of ovulation and are reduced in women approaching menopause when ovulation occurs less frequently *(Figure 1.4)*.

Figure 1.4 Ovulatory cycle: progesterone peak after ovulation disappears in anovular cycles just before menopause.

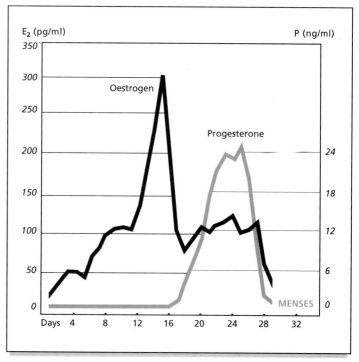

Inhibin suppresses synthesis of FSH (follicle-stimulating hormone) from the pituitary gland by a feedback mechanism, whereas activin stimulates it. The pituitary secretes FSH and LH (luteinising hormone) in response to activin and releasing hormones secreted from the hypothalamus in the central nervous system (CNS) *(Figure 1.5)*.

Figure 1.5 Negative and positive feedback systems between pituitary gland and ovaries.

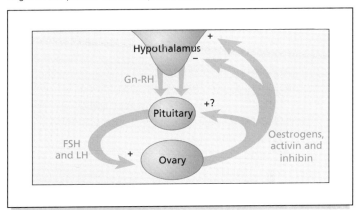

Reduction of oestrogen level at menopause is associated with increased outpouring of FSH and LH.

Age at menopause

This is determined by the number of ovarian follicles present in the ovaries. This declines from approximately 7,000,000 at birth to none after the menopause, but the number may vary as much as a hundred-fold in women of a given age range, e.g. 40-44 years (*Figure 1.6*).

Figure 1.6 Changes in germ cell numbers in the human ovary with increasing age.

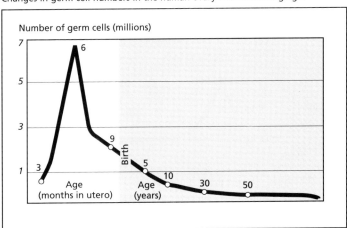

The average age at menopause is 51 years in industrialised societies. The most important factor in reducing the age at menopause is smoking. Observation of 2,570 American women for five years[7] found that smokers experienced a shift of about one and a half years advancement of the date of the menopause. Other possible factors are poor nutrition, nulliparity and low socio-economic status. It was thought that women from developing countries have an earlier menopause; this has not been confirmed by a cross-cultural survey of 400 women in seven countries[8]. It is possible that age at menopause reflects ageing and a late menopause is associated with a longer life span[9].

Menstrual cycle patterns

Menstrual cycles shorten as women reach their 40s, due to shortening of the follicular phase. Ageing follicles become less responsive to the effect of gonadotrophins. As women approach the menopause, the menses often become irregular and usually there are gaps of several months before they cease altogether (Figure 1.7). However, bleeding may recur, even after 12 months, due to renewed follicular activity. The menopausal transition starts with irregular menses around the age of 47.5 years and lasts for about 3.8 years, according to a recent prospective study of 2,570 women in Massachusetts[7].

Figure 1.7   The effect of age upon the interval between menstrual onsets.

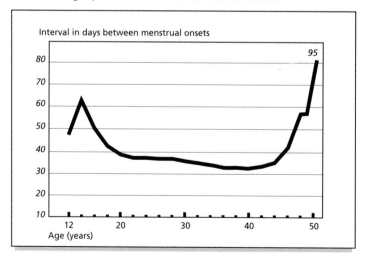

Hormone levels

As the menopause approaches, FSH levels rise steadily and LH levels increase around the age of 50. Serum inhibin and oestradiol levels fall.

During the menopause transition hormonal levels are extremely variable and this means that they are of poor predictive value with respect to timing of the menopause. This is particularly important with regard to predicting fertility.

Diagnosis of menopause

Some women who have menopausal blood levels of FSH and are diagnosed as 'menopausal' may revert to pre-menopausal status with low FSH and high oestradiol levels in subsequent months. From a practical viewpoint this implies the necessity of careful counselling on the need for contraception. Traditionally, this should be continued for two years after the date of the FMP in women under 50 years, and for one year in those over 50.

FSH levels

Serum FSH levels are commonly used to diagnose menopause, although tests may need to be repeated to avoid confusion from coincidence with the FSH peak in women who are still ovulating sporadically *(Table 1.1)*. By two to three years after the last menses, FSH increases to 10-15 times the premenopausal level. Usually 30 iu/l is taken as the cut-off point for diagnosis of menopause.

Table 1.1   **Reference ranges of female hormones (si units)**

Adult women	Oestradiol pmol/l	FSH iu/l	LH iu/l
Follicular	160 - 1,310	1 - 9	1 - 12
Ovulatory	900 - 2,290	6 - 26	16 - 104
Luteal	220 - 1,480	1 - 9	1 - 12
Post-menopausal	<100	30 - 118	16 - 66

From Department of Clinical Endocrinology, Birmingham and Midland Hospital for Women.

Levels of FSH and LH decrease with age and are negatively correlated with the body mass index.

Oestradiol

Oestrogen and progesterone levels decline dramatically in the last year before the last menstrual period (LMP). Serum oestradiol levels fall after the menopause to a level below 80 pmol/l compared with mean premenopausal levels of 550 pmol/l. These levels of oestradiol are difficult to measure, and there are methodological problems as low values are often below the sensitivity of the assay.

Although patients often request 'measurement of oestrogen levels', many laboratories are cautious about interpretation of results and the most appropriate use of oestradiol assay is in research. Ordinary clinical practice is better served by other tests, such as FSH or oestrone assay, although women on implants often need oestradiol levels measured.

Oestrone

Oestrone is the principal oestrogen circulating after the menopause. Average levels are about 100 pmol/l. It is formed from conversion of androstenedione and other precursors from the adrenal gland. The level of oestrone correlates positively with body mass index (*Figure 1.8*). Overweight women have higher levels of circulating oestrogen, greater bone density and a higher risk of uterine cancer than thin women because of the conversion in peripheral fat of androgenic precursors into oestrone (*Figure 1.9*).

Figure 1.8 Production rates of oestrone in micrograms per day plotted against weight in 34 post-menopausal women[10].

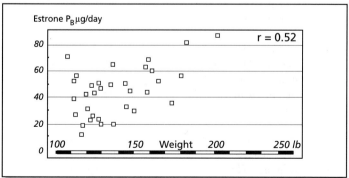

Reproduced with the permission of the authors and publisher.

Figure 1.9   The sources of oestrogen.

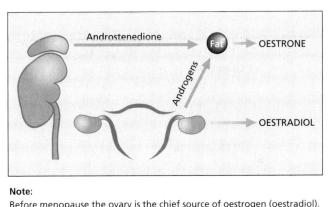

Note:
Before menopause the ovary is the chief source of oestrogen (oestradiol).
After menopause the adrenal gland is the chief source (oestrone by
conversion of androstenedione). Obese women convert adrenal androgens
more efficiently and have higher oestrone levels.

Androgens

Male hormones are important to women, and not only in the obvious
sense. Androgens enhance libido in both men and women (*Figure 1.10*).

The ovary is a major source of testosterone and androstenedione,
and following oophorectomy there is a 50% decrease in the serum
levels of both steroids. This may explain the dramatic fall in libido
which can be suffered by women whose ovaries have been removed
or irradiated.

A study of castrated Australian women who complained of loss of libido
attempted treatment with oestradiol implants[11]. These were unsuccessful
until they were supplemented by implants of testosterone. There was a
significant increase in sex drive in those who received both hormones
(*see Figure 1.10*).

After the natural menopause, the ovaries continue to secrete androgens
at a reduced level. The adrenal androgen dehydroepiandrosterone
sulphate (DHEAS) declines with age but is not affected by
menopause or HRT.

Figure 1.10 Effects of single initial implant of oestradiol and combined implant of testosterone and oestradiol on libido and sexual enjoyment (analogue scales) over 24 weeks. Arrow indicates time of insertion of testosterone implant in group, initially given oestradiol alone[11].

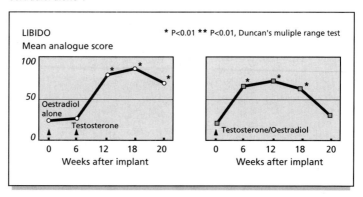

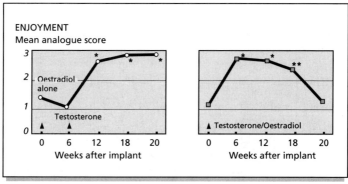

Reproduced with the permission of the author.

Sex hormone-binding globulin

Testosterone selectively binds to sex hormone-binding globulin (SHBG)[12]; only the unbound portion is free and physiologically active. This makes it difficult to measure, but some laboratories calculate a free testosterone index from total testosterone and SHBG assays. Endogenous and therapeutic oestrogen act on the liver to stimulate SHBG production so that oestrogen therapy always causes binding of testosterone and reduced levels of free testosterone (*Figures 1.11 and 1.12*).

Figure 1.11 Oestrogen increases hepatic synthesis of SHBG[13].

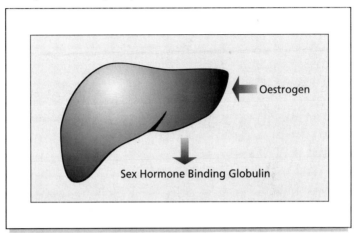

Reproduced with the permission of the author and publisher.

Figure 1.12 Sex hormone-binding globulin has a greater affinity for testosterone than oestradiol[13].

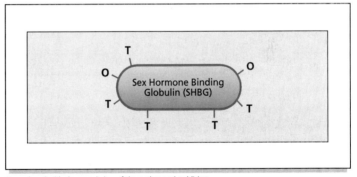

Reproduced with the permission of the author and publisher.

Conclusions

The physiology which underlies the menopause varies tremendously between individual women. The function of the adrenal and thyroid glands depends on adequate nutrition and stimulus, and the absence of disease; this affects women's health and the occurrence of symptoms. The post-menopausal ovaries supply small quantities of androgens and oestrogens, which are important for the health of older women *(Figure 1.13)*. Cigarette smoking reduces the level of circulating oestrogen and accelerates the onset of menopause.

Figure 1.13 Diagrammatic representation of the source of oestrogens in post-menopausal women[14].

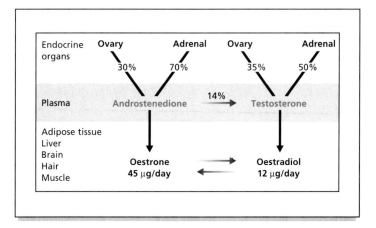

The date of the natural menopause can occur at any time over a span of 15 years and the premenopausal transition has a duration of over four years. Women's perception of symptoms changes according to their society and culture, negative images of menopause and their vulnerability following adverse life events. The underlying physiology remains approximately the same in women across the world and it is useful for the practice team to have an understanding of these changes.

References

1. World Health Organisation. Report of Study Group Geneva, 1994. (p9, fig 2.) In: Kanis JA, Pitt F. Epidemiology of Osteoporosis. *Bone* 1992; **31 (1)**: S7-15.

2. World Health Organisation. Report of Study Group, Geneva, 1994. (p13, fig 4). Cooper C, Campion G, Melton L. Hip fractures in the elderly: a worldwide projection. *Osteoporosis International* 1992; **2**: 285-9.

3. Department of Health. *Report of Advisory Group on Osteoporosis*. London: HMSO, November 1994.

4. Oliver MF, Boyd GS. Effect of bilateral ovariectomy on coronary-artery disease and serum-lipid levels. *Lancet* 1959; 690-3.

5. Wilkes HC, Meade TW. Hormone replacement therapy in general practice: a survey of doctors in the MRC's general practice research framework. *Br Med J* 1991; **302**: 1317-20.

6. Bernard Eskin MD, *The Menopause: comprehensive management, 2nd edition*. New York: McMillan NY 1988; 3-28.

7. McKinlay SM, Brambilla DJ, Posner JG. The normal menopause transition. *Am J Hum Biol*. 1992; **4**: 37-46.

8. Payer L. Menopause in various cultures. In: Bunger H, Boulet M (eds). *A portrait of the menopause*. Lancashire: Parthenon Publishing Group, 1991; 3-22.

9. Snowden DA *et al*. Is early natural menopause a biological marker of health and ageing? *Am J Pub Health* 1989; **79**: 709-14.

10. Longcope C, Jaffee W, Griffing G. Production rates of androgens and oestrogens in post-menopausal women. *Maturitas* 1981; **3**: 215-23.

11. Burger H, Hailes J, Nelson J. Effects of combined implants of oestradiol and testosterone on libido in post-menopausal women. *Br Med J* 1987; **294**: 936-7.

12. Anderson DC. Sex-hormone-binding globulin. *Clinic Educ* 1974; **3**: 69-96.

13. Coope J. *Hormone replacement therapy*. London: Royal College of General Practitioners, 1993.

14. Anderson ABM. *Human Reproductive Physiology*. Oxford: Blackwell Scientific Publications, 1979; 445.

CHAPTER **TWO**

Women's symptoms at the menopause and how to treat them

There has been a good deal of controversy about which symptoms are truly menopausal and related to changes in hormonal balance. Women and their families are only too ready to attribute to the menopause such symptoms as forgetfulness, tiredness and irritability. The application of a physical diagnostic label to these vague symptoms, which are common in both men and women, implies that they are easily treated with hormones and removes the obligation to probe further into possible social and psychological trigger factors and origins.

A postal survey of 1,120 women and 510 men in the Oxfordshire area was carried out by epidemiologists Bungay and Vessey[1]. Great care was taken not to implicate the menopause in the original questionnaire. In-depth questioning was then carried further in a second questionnaire to enquire about family, social and gynaecological problems. The graphs show the incidence of symptoms in men and women between the ages of 30 and 64 years (*Figure 2.1*).

Figure 2.1 Symptom patterns by age and sex, showing different types of responses[1].

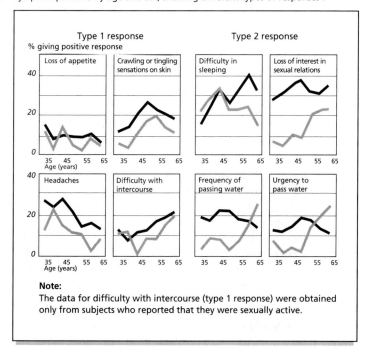

Note:
The data for difficulty with intercourse (type 1 response) were obtained only from subjects who reported that they were sexually active.

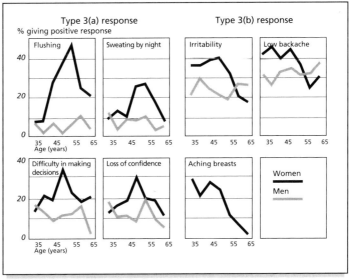

Reproduced with the permission of the authors.

Peaks of prevalence of night sweats, day sweats and flushing in women are clearly associated with the mean age of menopause. Less impressive peaks of loss of confidence and difficulty with decisions, which are probably associated with anxiety, appear just before the menopause. Insomnia goes on increasing into old age as does loss of sexual interest. The peak of anxiety-related symptoms just before the menopause does not necessarily mean that they are related to changes in hormone levels. Work by Hunter[2], a psychologist working with menopausal patients at Guy's Hospital, London, has shown that:

'...stereotyped beliefs about the menopause, assessed before the event, predicted depressed mood when the women became post-menopausal. Stereotype score was independent of current mood state. Negative beliefs could act as a filter through which physiological and emotional sensations are experienced, thus influencing women's perceptions and interpretations of the menopause. Mechanisms such as the labelling of bodily experiences and the attribution of symptoms may explain how this process might occur.

Those women who were already depressed before the menopause were also likely to be depressed during the climacteric. While this does not necessarily explain the increase in depression, depressed women might well anticipate the menopause more negatively and feel more helpless about it than others who are less depressed. If these negative views are held and the menopause is seen as yet another unpleasant and uncontrollable event, then any existing depression might be exacerbated.

In conclusion, these results are on the whole reassuring in that, apart from vasomotor symptoms and vaginal dryness, the menopause does not appear to have a major impact upon women's general health or their help-seeking behaviour. The incidence of hot flushes and vaginal dryness was lower than expected and both complaints also occurred, to a lesser extent, in premenopausal women.

Longitudinal findings replicate the cross-sectional results - despite the small size of the prospective sample. The main advantage of the longitudinal design is that symptoms reported by climacteric women can be interpreted in a broader context. The current study demonstrates the importance of assessing pre-existing levels of symptoms - as well as health beliefs, general health, life stress and health-related behaviour patterns such as exercise - when interpretations are made regarding the impact of the menopause upon the quality of women's lives.'

This longitudinal study is described in Chapter 3. Neither age nor time since menopause has been found to predict the hormone levels in an individual patient. Some women have high circulating oestrogen levels at an advanced age. However, nutrition is important and obesity increases the levels of both oestrone and oestradiol. Different ethnic groups have been studied. Mayan and Nigerian women have similar hormone levels to Caucasians. Rural Chinese women have lower levels of testosterone and oestradiol compared with British women of the same age. It is common for Western women to experience recurrence of flushes many years after the menopause, often as a response to stress, and this may reflect changes in endogenous oestrogen production.

Biological changes in the woman

In response to lower levels of circulating oestrogen, the uterus becomes smaller and if there are fibroids present these may shrink or become calcified. The lining of the womb (endometrium) becomes thinner and the breasts are reduced in size and are less vascular. Reduction in collagen thickness occurs in the skin and other tissues. All these changes are gradual and may take place over many years.

Hot flushes

Flushes occur as a result of vasomotor instability and often appear in the first few years before menopause in response to falling oestrogen levels. They are usually at a maximum in the year after the menopause, but may continue for many years afterwards in a sporadic manner.

Ginsburg has studied women during flushing episodes by measuring changes in hand and forearm blood flow. The onset of symptoms of the hot flush is associated with an immediate rise in blood flow to the hand and an increased pulse rate (*Figure 2.2*). No blood pressure changes occur and therefore the flush is not due to generalised release of a circulating vasodilator, but to localised vasodilatation in the skin

Figure 2.2 Peripheral blood flow in menopausal women who have hot flushes and those who do not[3]. Mean hand and forearm blood flow (mg/100 ml tissue/min) and pulse rate (beats/min) in six women before, during and after a menopausal hot flush.

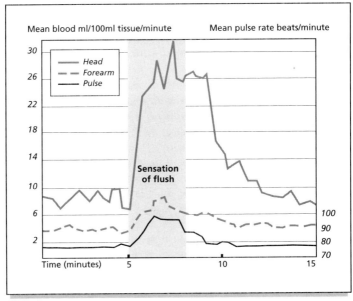

Reproduced with the permission of the authors and publisher.

of the face, neck and arms. A rise in skin temperature occurs after the flush and coincides with a fall in core temperature, which can be measured in the vagina or tympanic orifice.

No single hormone has been found to be responsible for flushes. It has been suggested that the hypothalamic thermoregulatory centre responds to a change in the body thermostat which reduces core temperature and sets off mechanisms to promote heat loss (flushes and sweats). Administration of a gonadotrophin-releasing hormone (Gn-RH) agonist may promote flushes. Three different substances (noradrenaline, dopamine and endogenous opioid peptides) have been identified as transmitters in animal studies, but are not confirmed by experiments in human subjects. Men also experience hot flushes after removal of the testes and it is possible that this is due to a similar mechanism. Some women never get hot flushes, others suffer excessively and can experience greatly reduced quality of life as their sleep is disturbed by nocturnal sweats. Menopausal flushes are abolished by sufficient dosage of oestrogen in nearly all women.

Effects of oestrogen on hot flushes

This was demonstrated by our double-blind, randomised, placebo-controlled, cross-over trial of 30 women taking *Premarin* 1.25 mg or placebo *(Figure 2.3)*. Despite large placebo responses the flushes showed a significantly greater response to oestrogen. It took two to three months to achieve the maximum effect of oestrogen and after the cross-over to placebo all the women experienced severe flushes (even those who had not suffered before the trial). These effects are probably due to the rise in SHBG which occurs due to the effect of oral oestrogen on hepatic synthesis. The globulin binds to oestrogen, delaying the full effect as the free active hormone is slowly released. After withdrawal of oestrogen, the SHBG slowly releases its store and the full effect of withdrawal is only felt after three months.

Oestrogen 'addiction'

This explains the occasional complaint of women that they are 'addicted to oestrogen'. Withdrawal of hormones causes falling serum levels and may precipitate severe flushing which always improves on re-taking the drug.

Figure 2.3 Effects of 'natural oestrogens' on menopausal symptoms and blood clotting[4]. Hot flushes in two groups of 15 women taking *Premarin* 1.25 or placebo in a double-blind cross-over trial[4].

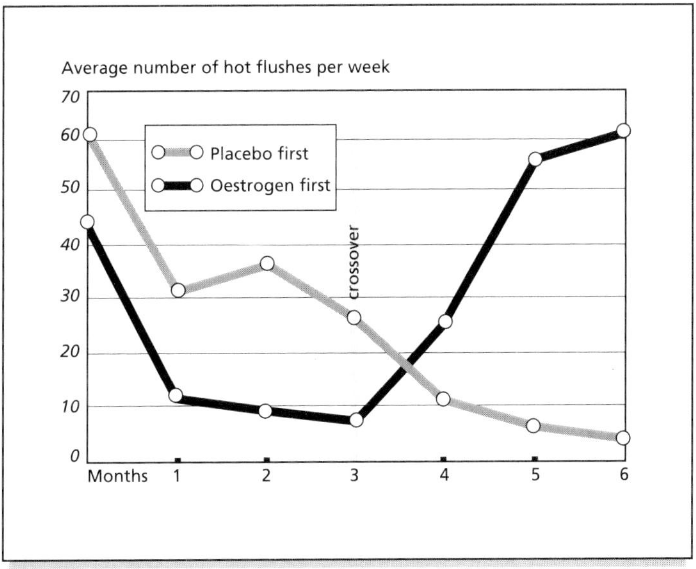

Reproduced with the permission of the authors and publisher.

Factors affecting flushing

Temperature

The temperature of the environment affects flushes. *Figure 2.4* shows the flushes in 25 women in the hot summer of 1976 - they recorded numbers of daily flushes and an observer recorded the maximum and minimum daily temperature. There was a highly significant correlation between the ambient temperature and the severity of flushes. This means that the recommendation to wear cool clothes and reduce room heating are not really old wives' tales - the cold shower treatment really works.

Exercise

A controlled study of 1,600 post-menopausal women in Sweden showed that flushes and sweats were only half as common in those who were physically active. *Figure 2.5* shows the reduction of 'vegetative symptoms', i.e. flushes, in physically active women aged 52-54 when compared with the general population.

Figure 2.4 A study of the effectiveness of propranolol in menopausal hot flushes[5]. (Propranolol was found to be no more effective than placebo so, in effect, the women were untreated). Relationship between number of flushes and temperature.

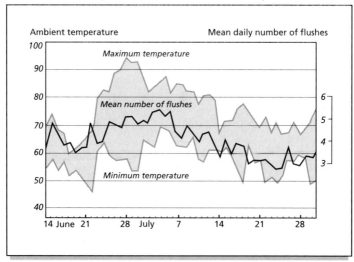

Reproduced with the permission of the authors and publisher.

Figure 2.5 Non-hormonal management of the menopause[6]. Moderate to severe vegetative symptoms among non-selected 52- to 54-year-old women and physically active post-menopausal women in Linköping, Sweden.

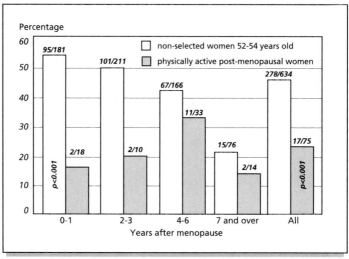

Reproduced with the permission of the author and publisher.

Psychological treatment

Cognitive-behavioural therapy, including training in relaxation, has been shown to reduce the incidence of flushes. This work is in progress at the clinic for menopausal patients at Guy's Hospital, London, under Hunter[2].

Evening primrose oil

No effect on flushing was observed which was any better than placebo, when a randomised, double-blind study was carried out on 56 flushing menopausal women in Stoke-on-Trent, UK. They took either capsules of EP 4g daily or placebo[7].

Paced respiration (deep breathing)

This has been shown by objective methods to reduce flushing.

Vaginal changes

After the menopause the vaginal epithelium becomes atrophic in some women, but this is by no means universal. A study of vaginal cytology by two doctors working at well-woman clinics and hospital outpatient clinics in London surveyed the vaginal smears of 148 women aged 45-82 years. They found that even over the age of 80 some women had well oestrogenised smears *(Figure 2.6)*. On the other hand, some younger women showed cytological evidence of severe oestrogen lack. Symptom questionnaires to patients found no difference in symptoms between women with vaginal atrophy and those with normal smears. This may be because menopausal symptoms occur in response to falling levels of oestrogen rather than to the chronic long-term level which is reflected by vaginal cytology.

Vaginal cytology is not a sufficiently sensitive test to be used for the initial assessment of menopausal women and their need for oestrogen.

Vaginal examination

In clinical practice, the state of the vagina is obvious to the examining doctor who attempts to obtain a cervical cytology specimen. The atrophic vagina is small, tender and bleeds easily, and a speculum is inserted with difficulty. The patient may admit to problems with sexual intercourse and can be reassured that local oestrogen therapy or HRT by any route are both highly effective treatments. Continuing sexual intercourse protects women against vaginal atrophy[9].

Figure 2.6 Cytological oestrogen assessment in the post-menopause according to age[8].

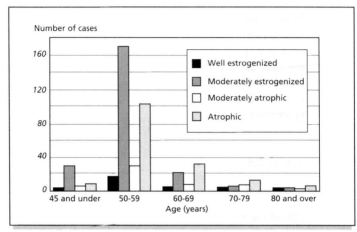

Reproduced with the permission of the author.

Urological symptoms

Over a quarter of the population of women past the menopause suffer from some kind of urinary problem, such as incontinence, pain on micturition, urgency or nocturia. Various attempts have been made to assess their response to hormonal treatment:

- Stress incontinence does not respond to oestrogen better than to placebo[10].

- Urgency and painful micturition improve on oestrogen, and a controlled trial of intravaginal oestriol found that it reduced the recurrence of urinary tract infections after the menopause[11]. If women are going to undergo an operation for relief of stress incontinence, it is often worth giving oestrogen pre-operatively to increase the tone of vaginal and urethral muscles and the thickness of the mucosa.

- Women who wear a supportive vaginal ring pessary to prevent prolapse or incontinence are often helped by local oestrogen pessaries or cream which reduce the frequency of infection and unpleasant discharge.

Psychological symptoms and changes in bones and blood vessels which occur at the menopause will be discussed later.

Abnormal bleeding around the time of the menopause

Many women regard unusual bleeding as a 'normal' symptom of the menopause. Painful, irregular or heavy bleeding is extremely common; a survey of over 1,000 women in their homes in 1990 reported that 38% had painful periods and 31% heavy periods, and one-third had asked for medical help about this in the past four months. One in 12 women aged 30-49 consult their general practitioner each year with heavy menstrual bleeding, which represents 12% of all gynaecological referrals. Referrals are increasing yearly and result in about 25,000 hysterectomies annually for menorrhagia.

Definition of heavy menstrual bleeding = loss of 80 ml or more per cycle

90% of the population lose less than 80 ml blood per cycle (*Figure 2.7*).

Figure 2.7 Frequency distribution (%) of menstrual blood loss in several hundred women in Oxford before insertion of a intrauterine device. Mean menstrual loss is 33 ml; median loss is 32 ml[12].

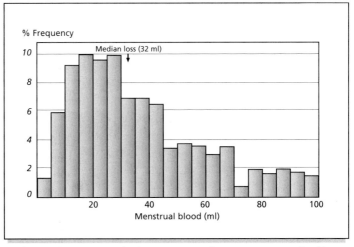

Reproduced with the permission of Oxford University Press from: Rees MCP. Menstrual problems. In: McPherson A (ed). Women's problems in general practice, 3rd Edition. Oxford: Oxford University Press, 1993.

Menorrhagia is thus defined as **menstrual blood loss of over 80 ml per cycle**. Many of the women who attend gynaecological clinics complaining of 'heavy bleeding' do not fall into this category, and objective measurement of blood loss shows that only 40% actually lose more than 80 ml per cycle. Rees[12] has measured this by soaking sanitary devices in 5% sodium hydroxide to convert blood to alkaline haematin and measuring its optical density. However, this method is only suitable for research. In actual clinical practice, full blood count, pelvic examination and vaginal ultrasound examination are the most useful tests. If the latter shows an abnormality, it is essential to refer to a gynaecologist for endometrial biopsy and/or hysteroscopy. Different methods of endometrial sampling, such as the Vabra or Pipelle devices are in use, and some women are admitted for dilatation and curettage (D&C) under anaesthesia. All these are methods of diagnosis, not treatment.

It is recommended that women under 40 should not undergo D&C as risks outweigh benefits.

The following conditions should be excluded before you decide that there is no organic pathology:

- Fibroids

- Endometrial pathology

- Blood dyscrasia and coagulation disorders

- Intrauterine device (IUD)

- Hypothyroidism

Diagnosis of heavy bleeding

It is a woman's perception of this which leads her to consult a doctor and may lead on to gynaecological referral. Women do not always have lower haemoglobin after a heavy bleed, but the presence of hypochromic anaemia should alert the general practitioner to its possibility, particularly if a full blood count shows the presence of reticulocytes. Vaginal examination may be followed by vaginal ultrasound examination to detect the presence of fibroids and check endometrial thickness.

Irregular bleeding, involving totally irregular periods, bleeding after intercourse or post-menopausal bleeding, should be investigated.

Vaginal ultrasound examination

A survey of over 1,000 Swedish women concluded that endometrial double thickness of <4 mm indicated a very low risk of malignancy. Over 8 mm thickness warrants further investigation by endometrial biopsy and/or hysteroscopy.

Why do women bleed excessively?

Progesterone levels are greatly reduced in women over 40 and, in the absence of ovulation, a progressive rise in oestrogen secretion causes endometrial proliferation without secretory change. The thickened endometrium breaks off and bleeds, sometimes in an uncontrolled manner, resulting in excessive blood loss.

Management of heavy bleeding

Blood count and other tests are essential to make a diagnosis and to verify the severity of bleeding.

Reassurance

This is important and the effectiveness of counselling is being currently evaluated in a randomised, controlled trial in Oxford.

Medical treatment

- **Mefenamic acid** has been shown to reduce blood loss and can be given during menstruation only (500 mg t.i.d.). Experimental evidence suggests that it transforms haemostatic plugs and reduces the number of vessels without a plug.

- **Tranexamic acid** 1.0-1.5 mg 8-hourly during menstruation is effective but should not be used in women with a history of thrombosis.

- **Danazol** is highly effective in the treatment of menorrhagia and also endometriosis. It is taken continuously, 200-400 mg daily. It has immunosuppressive properties and also acts on the hypothalamic-pituitary axis. Some women complain of acne and weight gain due to its androgenic properties, but others feel extremely well and it is worth a trial.

• Progestogens	are popular but there is little evidence as to their effectiveness. They are useful in producing regular cycles, a typical regime being norethisterone 5 mg t.i.d. days 19-26.
• Gestrinone	is effective but expensive.
• LH-RH analogues	are effective by producing a medical menopause which is reversible. Side-effects include hot flushes and loss of bone density.
• Oral contraceptives	are extremely effective in producing regular, controlled bleeds and have recently been licensed for use up to and beyond the age of menopause in healthy, non-smoking women.
• Progestogen-releasing intrauterine device	There is evidence that this is effective and it is now licensed for use in the UK as a contraceptive.

Surgical treatment

Hysterectomy is common and over 74,000 operations are carried out annually in Great Britain. It can be performed through an incision in the abdomen or the vagina and recently via laparoscopy. One or both ovaries may be removed during the operation. If both ovaries are removed before the menopause this substantially reduces the risk of breast cancer. However, the patient becomes more vulnerable to osteoporotic fracture and heart disease, and life expectancy is reduced by over five years if she does not take hormone therapy. Since many women do not comply with long-term therapy, it should not be routine practice to remove healthy ovaries during hysterectomy.

Endometrial ablation or resection involves a shorter operation and a shorter stay in hospital. Patients are able to return to work more quickly and there are fewer post-operative complications. Randomised, controlled trials have compared the outcome of abdominal hysterectomy with these new treatments; *Table 2.1* shows the results of the largest trial from Aberdeen.

Table 2.1   The Aberdeen study[13]

Treatment	Abdominal hysterectomy	Endometrial ablation or resection
Study size	99	105
Follow-up time	12 months	12 months
Process of care:		
-Operating time (median mins)	61	45 (mean)
-Length of stay (median days)	7	3 (mean)
Post-op complications	47%	15%
Duration of analgesia (median weeks)	1 - 2	<1
No pain at seven days	–	–
Time to resume daily activities (median weeks)	8 - 12	2 - 4
Menstrual outcomes:		
-No bleeding	100%	22%
-Light bleeding	–	62%
-Menstrual pain	–	–
Pelvic pain	13%	–
Emotional outcomes:		
-GHQ score <25%	26%	29%
Satisfaction:		
-Very satisfied with improvement	89%	78%
-Insufficient improvement	5%	6%
Re-operation rate	–	16% - 12 month

Women's attitudes

About 20% of Western women do not suffer from hot flushes, 20% suffer severely enough to consult a doctor and the rest do not. A postal survey of London women in the early 1970s showed that most women view the menopause with relief as periods cease and there is no need for contraception. Much more recent longitudinal studies in Britain and abroad confirm these early conclusions and are dealt with more fully in the section on psychological symptoms (see Chapter 5).

Contraception over the age of 40

Although fertility is considerably reduced at this age, couples still make mistakes and there are many thousands of unexpected and unwanted pregnancies in older women.

Table 2.2 **Pregnancies in women over 45 England and Wales per annum**

	Number 1993	Rate per 1,000 women aged 45 - 49	Number 1994	Rate per 1,000 women aged 45 - 49
Live births	539	0.3	488	0.3
Abortions	494	0.28	440	0.24

From OPCS Monitor Series AB

It is important to survey contraceptive methods in women with a uterus attending a mid-life clinic. The diagnosis of pregnancy can be difficult and a spell of amenorrhoea in a woman in her mid-40s may be due to:

• Pregnancy

• Effect of progestogen contraception

• Menopause

• Prolactinoma

• Effect of drugs, anorexia nervosa, endocrine illness

Menopause is diagnosed by raised FSH/LH levels, negative pregnancy test and possibly ultrasound examination to exclude pregnancy. Some women 'go in and out of the menopause' and a period of amenorrhoea with menopausal levels of FSH/LH may be followed by a bleed and normal gonadotrophin levels. It is essential to continue contraception until one year after LMP in women over 50 and two years after LMP in younger women.

Sterilisation

This is becoming a popular choice for older couples. Careful counselling is necessary. A woman who has completed her family is often a better candidate than her husband who may wish to father a child later in life if the partnership does not survive. Female sterilisation is effective (failure rate 1 in 500 as an interval procedure) and is safe. There are no reported long-term physical sequelae. It can be performed under local or general anaesthetic with fallopian tubal patency interrupted by diathermy, surgery, clips or rings.

One in three couples in the UK using contraception choose this method and more than 60 million women are sterilised worldwide. Vasectomy is performed under local anaesthetic and is a safe, simple and effective procedure (early failure rate one in 1,000, late failure rate one in 3,000). From time to time some long-term serious side-effects, such as increased risk of cardiovascular disease, prostatic and testicular cancer, have been suggested but as yet these have not been substantiated.

Combined oral contraceptives

For healthy, non-smoking women the 'pill' provides cheap, effective and convenient contraception which is now recognised as safe until after the menopause (FDA Guidelines).

Around the age of 52-4 many pill-users may prefer to switch to long-term HRT plus a barrier method for a couple of years. The combined oral contraceptive (COC) provides protection against loss of bone density but probably not against heart disease. Many women stopping the pill notice that they suffer from flushes and these also occur during the pill-free interval when oestrogen levels are falling. The COC reduces the incidence of ovarian and endometrial cancer and drastically minimises the heavy bleeding of menorrhagia, producing predictable, manageable 'periods'.

Choice of preparation

Recent advice from the Committee on the Safety of Medicines (CSM) warns against using oral contraceptives containing the progestogens, gestodene or desogestrel, because of an increased risk of venous thrombosis. A change of pill is advised unless the patient is unwilling to change, having experienced problems with other brands. For medicolegal reasons, it is useful to record the fact that you have consulted the patient and that this is her choice. Immediate transfer is advised at the end of the pack, without a pill-free interval. Although this is now official CSM policy, countries other than the UK and Germany are more sceptical about the risk of using these new progestogens. The risk of venous thromboembolism can be usefully expressed as:

- Healthy women not taking
  progestogens   5 of 100,000 each year.

- Women in the year of a pregnancy   60 of 100,000 each year.

- Women taking combined pills
  containing gestodene
  or desogestrel   30 of 100,000 each year.

- Women taking combined pills
  containing levonorgestrel,
  norethisterone, ethynodiol diacetate   15 of 100,000 each year.

- The mortality of venous thromboembolic disease is 2%.

It will be seen that the risk of fatality is extremely low.

Further advice may be obtained from the following addresses:

Faculty of Family Planning and Reproductive Health Care
Royal College of Obstetricians and Gynaecologists
27 Sussex Place
London NW1 4RG
Telephone: 0171-724 2441

The Family Planning Association

27-35 Mortimer Street

London W2N 7RJ

Telephone: 0171-636 7866

Progestogen-only or 'mini-pill'

This is a useful alternative at any age and may cause amenorrhoea.

Emergency contraception

The morning-after (or later) pill works up to 72 hours after intercourse and even after that it is worth trying. Two tablets of a high-dose 50 µg pill such as *Ovran* are taken as soon as possible and repeated 12 hours later.

Insertion of a copper IUD is effective up to five days after intercourse and is useful if there has been multiple exposure. Contraindications to high-dose oestrogen are a history of DVT, jaundice, porphyria, sickle-cell disease and **current** focal migraine. In the future, mifepristone will probably be used. It is effective but awaits a license.

The intrauterine device (IUD)

This can be checked and left *in situ* until one year after menopause (it is usually removed then because of cervical stenosis preventing removal in some older women). *Multiload Cu 375* is one of the most commonly used devices in the UK. It lasts for five years. The pregnancy rate is approximately 2/100 women years, about 5% of these being ectopic pregnancies.

A recent development is the levonorgestrel IUD which delivers levonorgestrel 10 µg daily into the endometrium, avoiding unwanted systemic effects. It is licensed for three years' use but this should shortly be extended to five years. It is extremely effective in reducing heavy bleeding and reduces the risk of infection. With a failure rate of only 0.2%, it acts in the usual manner of progestogen, changing cervical mucus and making the endometrium less receptive to a fertilised ovum. Its use is not associated with ectopic pregnancy. Slight spotting may occur in the early months of use.

Figure 2.8 The levonorgestrel intra-uterine device.

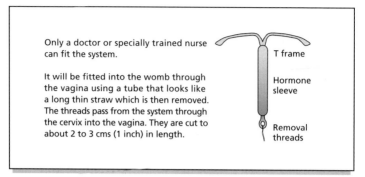

Only a doctor or specially trained nurse can fit the system.

It will be fitted into the womb through the vagina using a tube that looks like a long thin straw which is then removed. The threads pass from the system through the cervix into the vagina. They are cut to about 2 to 3 cms (1 inch) in length.

T frame

Hormone sleeve

Removal threads

Injectable progestogens

Depo-Provera (medroxyprogesterone acetate) is effective for 12 weeks and is useful for women who cannot take oestrogen or who may forget to take the pill. It causes anovulation and may lower oestrogen levels - two studies showed reduced bone density in long-term users. Many users have amenorrhoea. It is worth checking serum oestradiol levels and if these are below 100 pmol/l on two occasions oestrogen can be prescribed in addition. The World Health Organisation (WHO) Collaborative Study on Neoplasia and Steroid Contraceptives concluded that this preparation has no effect on the rates of ovarian, cervical or breast cancer but greatly reduces the incidence of endometrial cancer

The 'double Dutch' method

Barrier methods can be used in addition to hormonal methods in high-risk couples (e.g. recent change of partner) or instead of hormones in monogamous partnerships. Female or male condoms protect against STD and AIDS. The flat spring diaphragm, spring diaphragm or cervical cap needs to be fitted and used together with a spermicide.

Natural family planning

There is extreme variation in cycle length in the perimenopause, with cycles varying from two to 16 weeks and over in length. This renders the use of the so-called 'safe period' even more difficult and unsafe than in younger women.

Sexual problems in middle age

A recent survey of couples aged 40 to 70 showed that a substantial number were suffering from unsatisfactory sexual relationships, and 25% of men were impotent at the age of 65. Levels of androgen fall with advancing age and this reduces erectile efficiency. Many men are affected by heavy drinking or smoking, drugs to treat blood pressure or prostate problems, or diseases such as diabetes or heart disease. Impotence among men with diabetes ranges from 30-50% and sometimes impotence is complained of as a problem before the doctor has diagnosed that the patient has diabetes. Medical help is needed. Self-injection with medications such as alprostadil is often effective, and another possibility is the use of an appliance to help maintain an erection. Referral to a genitourinary specialist is helpful.

In discussing sexuality, which is obviously a function of a couple rather than a single person, male erectile dysfunction has been mentioned first. This is because it is probably more important than female problems, such as vaginal atrophy or lack of lubrication. Sexual problems occur frequently at and after the menopause and it is common for a difficulty to be blamed on the woman's menopause. However, an American survey of couples over the age of 45 demonstrated that the most important factor in maintaining a good sex life after the menopause is the quality of sex before the menopause. A survey of women attending a gynaecological clinic showed that those who had continued to have sexual intercourse had larger, more elastic vaginas and fewer problems with atrophy than those who had ceased to have sex[9]. No difference in hormone levels was found, except that the sexually functioning group had higher androgen levels. This may have been either cause or effect. Women with higher androgen levels have higher libido (see Chapter 1) and probably more frequent sex. Sexual intercourse may increase testosterone levels in the woman, either by absorption from semen through the vaginal wall, or by stimulation of ovarian and adrenal function.

There is little doubt that the menopause *per se* affects sexual function. Vaginal dryness and atrophy can occur due to low oestrogen levels and are treated by lubricants, *Replens* application, or local or systemic oestrogen. Women who have abstained from sex for some time and have started a new relationship may find sex painful and should be offered HRT.

Premature menopause

Early loss of fertility may be compensated for by ovum donation in selected couples. Hormonal manipulation is essential and there is a nationwide shortage of donor eggs. Further information is available from the London Gynaecology and Fertility Centre.

Conclusions

Physical changes in the vagina and urethra may give rise to troublesome symptoms which often respond to local or systemic hormone therapy. Women need advice on contraception and help in dealing with sexual difficulties. Encouragement to tackle the diverse manifestations of social and family dysfunction, and education about questions of preventive health, are appropriately offered in general practice. Hormone therapy can only be part of the answer. The menopause is an important event. The immediate symptoms are often negligible and do not threaten the woman's health, although they may create considerable anxiety. However, silent changes which occur gradually in blood vessels and bones increase the risk of heart disease and fractures, and it is these which justify hormone replacement therapy (HRT) in many women. Careful balancing of risks and benefits, and individual counselling, are called for from the primary health-care team. Hormonal and non-hormonal treatments are available for menopausal symptoms after diagnosis has been achieved[14].

References

1. Bungay GT, Vessey MP, McPherson CK. Study of symptoms in middle life with special reference to the menopause. Br Med J 1980; **281**: 181-3.

2. Hunter M. The South-East longitudinal study of the climacteric and post-menopause. Maturitas 1992; **14** (2): 117-26.

3. Ginsburg J, Hardiman P, O'Reilly P. Cardiovascular responses during the menopausal hot flush. Br Med J 1989; **298**: 1488-9.

4. Coope J, Thomson J. Effect of 'natural' oestrogens on menopausal symptoms and blood clotting. Br Med J 1975; **4**: 139-143.

5. Coope J, Williams S, Patterson JS. A study of the effectiveness of propranolol in menopausal hot flushes. Br J Obstet & Gynaecol 1978; **85**: 472-5.

6. Notelovitz M. Non-hormonal management of the menopause. In: Berg G, Hammar M (eds). *Modern management of the menopause*. Carnforth: Parthenon Publishing Group, 1994; 513-23.

7. Chenoy R, Hussain S, Taylor U *et al*. Effect of oral gamolenic acid from evening primrose oil on menopausal flushing. *Br Med J* 1994; **308**: 501-3.

8. Gordon H. Cytological estrogen assessment in the post menopause according to age. In: Campbell S (ed). *The management of the menopause and post-menopause*. p 264.

9. Leiblum S, Bachmann G. The sexuality of the climacteric woman. In: Eskin BA (ed). *The menopause: comprehensive management 2nd Edition*. New York: Macmillan Publishing Co; 2988.

10. Cardozo L. Role of estrogens in the treatment of female urinary incontinence. *J Am Geriat Soc* 1990; **38**: 326-8.

11. Raz R, Stamm WE. A controlled trial of intra-vaginal estriol in post-menopausal women with current urinary tract infections. *New Engl J Med* 1993; **329**: 802-3.

12. Rees MCP. Heavy painful periods. In: Drife JO (ed). *Clinical obstetrics & gynaecology: dysfunctional uterine bleeding and menorrhagia Vol 2*. London: Balliere Tindall, 341-56.

13. Pinion S *et al*. Randomised trial of hysterectomy, endometrial laser ablation, and transcervical endometrial research for dysfunctional uterine bleeding. *Br Med J* 1994; **309**: 979-83.

14. Coope J. Hormonal and non-hormonal interventions for menopausal symptoms. *Maturitas* 1996; **23**: 159-68.

CHAPTER **THREE**

Why women do or don't take HRT

Why women take HRT

Prevention of osteoporosis

This is important to women after the menopause. A 50-year-old white woman has a 15% lifetime chance of hip fracture, 32% for vertebral fracture and 15% for Colles' fracture. In fractures occurring before the age of 75, loss of bone density is probably the most important risk factor. After this age the use of sedatives, poor nutrition and a dangerous environment precipitate falling, but fragile bones contribute to the risk.

World Health Organisation definition of osteoporosis (1994)

'A disease characterised by low bone mass and microarchitectural deterioration of bone tissue, leading to enhanced bone fragility and a consequent increase in fracture risk.'

The WHO defined categories of osteoporosis in terms of bone density. The reduced bone densities referred to in this definition are in relation to the young adult mean value.

- Normal: a value for bone mineral density (BMD), or bone mineral content (BMC), within 1 SD of the young adult reference mean.

- Low bone mass: (osteopenia)   individuals with values reduced by more than 1 SD below the young adult mean, but less than 2.5 SD below this value have 'low bone mass (osteopenia)'.

- Osteoporosis: individuals with values 2.5 SD or more below the young adult mean have 'osteoporosis'. Individuals with fragility fractures and osteoporosis have 'severe osteoporosis'.

Low bone density has no symptoms and is not a disease *per se*, but it is the most important risk factor for fractures. Improvement of bone density prevents fracture. In the UK there are 60,000 hip, 50,000 wrist and 40,000 diagnosed vertebral fractures every year and the incidence is increasing across the world (*see Figures 1.1 and 1.2*).

Peak bone mass is achieved in young adult life and is influenced by date of menarche, whether a girl has amenorrhoea, smoking habit, lack of exercise and dietary calcium; genetic factors are also important. At the menopause the bone density is reduced at the rate of 1-3% per year as bone resorption exceeds the formation of new bone. This can be prevented by taking oestrogen in sufficient dosage for a long period, probably 7-10 years post-menopause. Even this duration of therapy may have little effect after the age of 75, when fracture risk increases. Women who are at high risk (e.g. family history, use of corticosteroids) should continue with HRT if possible throughout life. Those who sustain an osteoporotic fracture may be well advised to start HRT at a later age as it is effective after 70 years.

The following is advice to women over 40 years of age that should be displayed in the waiting area.

CHUSE to prevent osteoporosis:

Calcium...........................Eat more (at least 1,000 mg daily)

Hormones..........................Try them - ask your doctor

Ultraviolet sunlight.........15 minutes daily outdoors

Smoking ....Cut down or STOP!

Exercise ....Get going

CHUSE illustrates the measures which have been shown to be effective by large population studies or clinical experiments. **Calcium intake** is important throughout life, particularly in childhood, during pregnancy and after the menopause. Placebo-controlled studies have shown that calcium supplements are more effective than placebo in maintaining bone density after the menopause. In women just past the menopause oestrogen is much more efficacious than calcium. Older women need encouragement to take enough calcium in the diet (see protocol for health education clinics) and to supplement with calcium gluconate, citrate or other salts if necessary.

Oestrogen therapy is the most effective preventive treatment and protects bone density at all sites. It should be taken in sufficient dosage (see Chapter 2) and works by implant, orally or transdermally.

43

Ultraviolet light acts on the skin to synthesise vitamin D, which is then stored in the liver in an altered form and released as necessary for the formation of new bone. Vitamin D is essential to the absorption of dietary calcium. Short exposure of face and hands in the open air each day is sufficient for most people. A controlled French survey of housebound elderly patients in a nursing home demonstrated that adding vitamin D and calcium supplements to their diet reduced the incidence of hip fracture in the treated group[1].

Smoking reduces the effect of HRT by increasing the role of liver enzymes in conjugating and destroying oestrogen. Heavy smokers are more likely to have an early menopause and are more at risk from fractures.

Exercise protects bone health by increasing muscle pull and stimulating new bone formation. Tennis players have greater bone density in the arm which holds the racquet. A controlled study showed that women rowers had greater spinal bone density than a control group who did not row. Weight-bearing exercise is particularly valuable and space exploration has been shown to cause rapid osteoporosis in astronauts. Stroke patients suffer loss of bone density in the hemiplegic limbs.

Diagnosis of low bone density

Table 3.1 shows the main risk factors for osteoporosis.

Table 3.1	**Risk factors for osteoporosis[2]**	
	Endogenous	*Exogenous*
	Female sex	Low body weight
	Post-menopausal status	Premature menopause
	Caucasian race	Corticosteroid therapy
	Family history	Cigarette smoking
		Alcohol consumption
		Prolonged immobility
		Malabsorption
		Thyrotoxicosis
		Hyperparathyroidism

Reproduced with the permission of the author and publisher.

Alcohol is harmless and may increase bone density if taken in moderate amounts (up to two units daily). Heavy drinking is associated with fractures probably due to a combination of factors such as poor dietary calcium, increased risk of falls and altered liver metabolism.

Diagnosis of spinal fractures by X-ray is useful in older women with chronic back pain. Densitometry is available in many centres (*Table 3.2*). DEXA is dual energy X-ray absorptiometry and is quick and safe with low exposure to X-rays. The patient does not need to undress. Quantitative computed tomography (QCT) is accurate, but has greater X-ray exposure; it takes about 20 minutes and so is difficult for very ill patients.

Table 3.2   **Clinical indications for bone densitometry**[3]

Clinical findings	Objectives
Oestrogen deficiency - (particularly after early natural or surgical menopause, prolonged amenorrhoea, or where critical in decision about HRT).	Selective case findings
Vertebral deformity, multiple low trauma fractures or osteopenia noted on X-rays.	Confirm diagnosis
Monitoring therapy Long-term corticosteroid use (more than 5 mg daily is thought to be deleterious to bone).	Quantify response Identify fast bone losers
Other forms of secondary osteoporosis (anorexia nervosa, alcohol abuse, hyperparathyroidism, thyrotoxicosis, hypogonadism, malabsorption syndrome, post-gastrectomy and myeloma).	Quantify bone loss

Treatment of low bone density

Hormone replacement therapy is extremely effective. Bleed-free forms are popular with older women as they do not cause 'periods'. Men and women who do not wish to take hormones can be treated with biphosphonates. Etidronate is used for those who already have spinal fractures and also for prevention. Alendronate does not cause the mineralisation defect caused by etidronate if used for prolonged periods. Others (tilodronate, pamidronate, clodronate and risedronate) may come to market in the next few years. Anabolic steroids cause weight gain and fluid retention and are not used widely in the UK.

Oestrogens protect against heart disease

Figure 3.1 shows the causes of death in women aged 45-74 years, taken from data obtained from the OPCS (Office of Population Censuses and Surveys) in 1992 in Great Britain. As British women have an average age at death of over 80 years all these deaths can be regarded as premature. Nearly 30,000 premature deaths from heart disease occur each year in British women. Many of these could be prevented by reducing smoking in young women and educating children about the risk. Long-term use of HRT in older women would also reduce cardiac deaths. Ischaemic heart disease is twice as likely to occur after the menopause. When groups of women of similar age are compared the premenopausal group have half the incidence of coronary heart disease compared with those who are post-menopausal. Before the menopause, endogenous oestrogen protects women from heart disease. There is a steep rise in heart attacks in women after middle age and equal incidence in men and women after the age of 80.

Figure 3.1   Mortality in women aged 45-74 years.

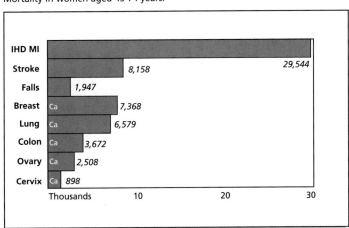

Heart disease is under-diagnosed in women. Exercise electrocardiograms are more likely to give misleading results, and women are more likely to die as a result of cardiac surgery because the disease is diagnosed at a later stage.

Oestrogen protects the heart and the arteries. A number of large population studies have examined the risk of developing symptoms or of dying from heart disease, and women who are taking oestrogen have a 40% reduction in risk compared with non-users (*Figure 3.2*)[4,5].

Figure 3.2   The incidence of death caused by heart disease in women taking or not taking HRT[6].

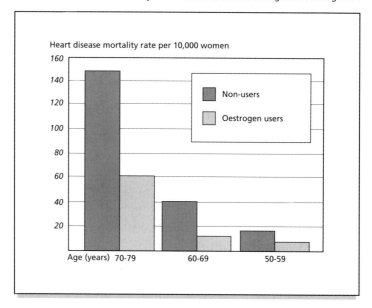

There is considerable argument about this, as it is known that women who are already healthy, of higher social class and less likely to smoke are more likely to take HRT (see Chapter 7 and discussion of randomised, controlled trials).

Nevertheless, all the epidemiological studies point in the same direction, i.e. the protective effect of oestrogen. HRT not only protects healthy women who are less likely to develop heart disease, but can be given to women who already have proven coronary disease. Survival is increased in HRT users (*see Figure 3.3*).

Figure 3.3   Ten-year survival of patients with left main coronary stenosis of 50% or greater, or other stenosis of 70% or greater.

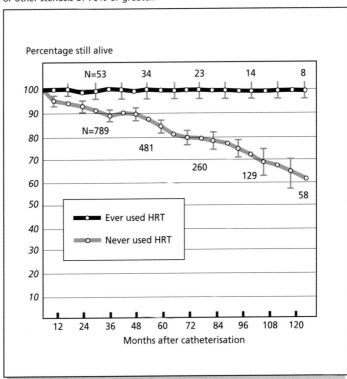

It is possible that a randomised, controlled trial will show that oestrogen is protective but that the actual amount of protection may be reduced from 40% to a lower level.

Experimental evidence confirms the conclusions of population studies. Observation of cynomolgus monkeys (which resemble human females in as far as they experience a similar menstrual cycle) by a group in the United States has shown that those animals which are given oestradiol develop smaller plaques in the coronary vessels than the untreated group. As we can see from *Figure 3.4*, the addition of progesterone does not significantly reduce the protective effect of oestrogen.

Figure 3.4   In surgically post-menopausal cynomolgus monkeys, both oestradiol and oestradiol plus progesterone therapy decreased coronary artery atherosclerotic plaque development without increasing plasma concentrations of HDL cholesterol.

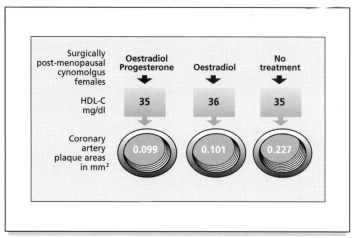

From: Adams et al. Inhibition of coronary artery atherosclerosis by 17-beta estradiol in ovariectomized monkeys. Lack of an effect of adding progesterone. Arteriosclerosis 1990: 10: 1051-7.

Clinical experiments

Cardiac catheterisation is used to study the condition of the coronary arteries in symptomatic women, and over 80% reduction in coronary artery disease has been observed in women taking oestrogen therapy. Normal coronary arteries and peripheral arteries dilate when exposed to acetylcholine, but diseased arteries constrict. When oestradiol is given intravenously it restores the vasodilative effect of acetylcholine. Volterrani[7] has demonstrated the effect of sublingual oestradiol beta 1 mg in increasing blood flow in the forearm and reducing peripheral vascular resistance. A British group has shown the increase in arterial tone which occurs after menopause *(Figure 3.5 overleaf)* and demonstrated that transdermal oestradiol reduces the pulsatility index.

Effect on lipids

This ratio is important in patients at risk of coronary heart disease and atherosclerosis. Increased HDL and lowered LDL is beneficial and *vice versa.*

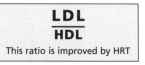

49

Figure 3.5 Correlation between baseline pulsatility index (PI) and time since menopause[8].

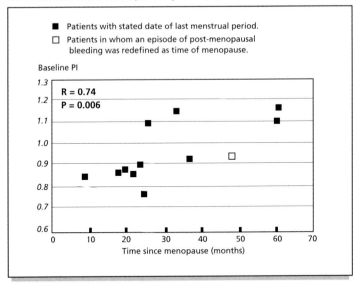

Reproduced with the permission of the authors and publisher.

Conjugated equine oestrogen increases triglycerides but oestrogen has a favourable effect on blood lipid pattern, increasing HDL, lowering LDL and reducing total cholesterol (*Figure 3.6*). Androgenic progestogens, such as norethisterone, antagonise some of these effects but this is less so with 'lipid-friendly' progestogens such as MPA (medroxyprogesterone acetate) and dydrogesterone. The effect of oestrogen is so marked that it overrides the effect of progestogen in women with a uterus who need to take both hormones. Oestrogen 'works' both orally or transdermally.

Lipid clinics recognise the beneficial effect of oestrogen and it is used as first-line therapy in some women. If necessary, specific lipid-lowering drugs such as the statins can be added later for increased effect. One of the case studies in Chapter 8 shows the effect of HRT in a woman of 60 with angina, abnormal lipid pattern and adverse family history.

Do oestrogens cause thrombosis?

This has been a vexed question ever since a group of women taking combined HRT containing mestranol developed more episodes of deep vein thrombosis than their non-treated controls. Clinical studies of

WHY WOMEN DO OR DON'T TAKE HRT

Figure 3.6 Effect of transdermal oestradiol patches in 52 women[9].

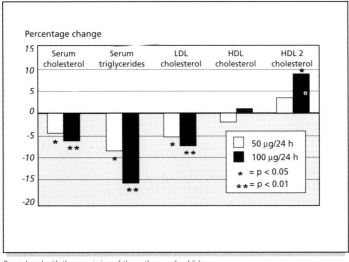

Reproduced with the permission of the authors and publisher.

men with prostate cancer have shown that the large doses of oestrogen used to treat their condition were associated with an increased incidence of deaths from thromboembolism. An early attempt to give preventive treatment to men who had suffered a myocardial infarct, by prescribing high doses of conjugated equine oestrogen (2.5-5.0 mg), was abandoned prematurely because the men in the treated groups showed an increased incidence of thrombosis[10]. However, women may react differently from men and the high doses of oestrogen used in these experiments are not commonly prescribed nowadays. More recent evidence is encouraging and suggests that there is no increased risk of thromboembolic disease with the doses and preparations of HRT which are currently in use at the menopause.

The Boston Collaborative Group Surveillance Program[11] employed nurse monitors to interview patients admitted to 24 general medical and surgical wards in 24 hospitals in one year. Census data were used to extrapolate findings on 5,339 patients to a population of 177,000 women aged 40-69 years. Altogether they identified only three cases of idiopathic venous thromboembolism out of an estimated 16,500 oestrogen users. This did not differ significantly from the incidence of 15 cases among an estimated 160,500 women aged 40-69 years

51

who were non-users. Non-idiopathic cases due to fracture, cancer, previous pulmonary embolism etc. were excluded in both groups. Further epidemiological surveys published in 1979 and 1983 showed that the incidence of phlebothrombosis was not significantly different in groups of oestrogen users and matched control patients[12].

Various randomised, controlled studies have examined the changes in blood coagulation which may occur in women using oestrogen, and compared these with the results from matched non-users. A variety of studies, with conflicting results, have been carried out using tests such as factor VII and X assay, antithrombin III and prothrombin time measurement. Our study of women using conjugated equine oestrogens, 1.25 mg[13], demonstrated significant increase of factors VII and X and shortened prothrombin time after three months' use, and acceleration of thrombin-induced platelet aggregation after a year. However, there was no increase in clinical thrombosis in patients taking oestrogen and it should be pointed out that the dose of oestrogen used was higher than that in current therapeutic use (0.625 mg).

Many studies have shown no change in coagulation factors on HRT and it is accepted that levels of plasma factors alone cannot predict a hypercoagulable state. Some recent studies have shown an increased risk of venous thromboembolism in women taking HRT[14]. The risk is still very small at an estimated three in 10,000 compared with one in 10,000 among those not taking HRT.

For most women after the menopause, the cardiovascular benefits of oestrogen therapy far outweigh the risk of thromboembolism. Unfortunately, fears of medicolegal proceedings and the current package inserts and data sheets which are in use by pharmaceutical companies act as a deterrent to the long-term use of hormone therapy.

It would be prudent to review the need for HRT in women with predisposing factors such as a personal or family history of thromboembolism, severe varicose veins, obesity, surgery, trauma or prolonged bed rest. Sometimes a surgeon or anaesthetist planning a risky operation, such as a hip replacement, may request abstinence from oestrogen therapy for a short period. These arrangements are open to negotiation between the individual patient and the unit concerned.

For most women, the small increase in risk of venous thromboembolism should be seen in the context of the benefits in treatment.

Relief of symptoms

Oestrogen, with or without progestogen, is highly effective in the relief of menopausal symptoms such as flushes, secondary insomnia and vaginal atrophy. These are dealt with more fully in Chapter Two. There is no doubt that for many women HRT improves their quality of life.

Summary

Preventive hormone therapy is here to stay and the recognition and treatment of vulnerable groups is work for general practitioners. The following passage is taken from Dewhurst's *Textbook of Obstetrics and Gynaecology* published in 1986[15]:

'Efforts need rather to be concentrated on the recognition and treatment of high risk subgroups of post-menopausal women such as women under 40 who have a premature menopause where benefit/cost ratios are unequivocal and treatment can be instituted effectively.

In the past the risks of oestrogen therapy have probably been overestimated and the benefits have been underestimated. With these considerations in mind, the following approach to hormone replacement may be advised:

1. Short-term hormone replacement and appropriate therapy should be given for specific menopausal symptoms (hot flushes, atrophic vaginitis etc.) for as long as symptoms persist;

2. Long-term hormone replacement should be given in all women under the age of 40 who are hypo-oestrogenic or undergo a spontaneous premature menopause or induced premature menopause;

3. Long-term hormone replacement should be given to any informed patient who requests it provided there are no contraindications and adequate continuing medical supervision is available. It is not ethically justifiable to withhold hormone replacement from fully informed patients who request it although all such patients must be assessed and managed on an individual basis.'

Why women do not take HRT

Breast cancer

Breast cancer affects one in 12 women in Britain, and the question of whether the risk is increased by hormone therapy is enormously important to women.

A recent editorial by McPherson in the *British Medical Journal*[16] points out that a 50-year-old woman faces the following lifetime risks:

- coronary heart disease   45%

- hip fracture   15%

- breast cancer   8%

Most of the meta-analyses to date measure the effect of oestrogen alone and show that long-term use of oestrogen (over 10 years) increases the risk of breast cancer, possibly by up to 50%, but shorter use does not affect risk.

It was hoped that added progestogen would protect oestrogen users against breast cancer but this has not proved to be the case, either in the Swedish study of 23,000 HRT users published in 1989[17], or the recent updated analysis of the on-going American study of the health of over 48,000 nurses[18]. In the Nurses' Health Study there was a 40% increase in the risk of breast cancer in women currently using HRT for over five years. A 70% increase occurred in older women aged 60-64 years. Reliable information is lacking on how long the increased risks continue after stopping treatment.

McPherson concludes:

'If the effects on breast cancer last rather longer than expected after, say, 10 years' use then hormone supplements could be responsible for an average net loss of years of life. If, secondly, the attributable effects of combined supplement on deaths from heart disease are rather less than currently expected after the supplements are stopped then longer use may also result in an aggregated net loss. Neither of these hypotheses is implausible. The balance with prevention of osteoporosis will then be further compromised, and cost-effectiveness will depend crucially on improved quality of life owing

> to relief of symptoms and prevention of fractures, to be set against a possible net loss of years of life. For women with a higher baseline risk of breast cancer, the symptom thresholds will then be more severe still. With the falling baseline risk of heart disease, the balance will move away from the prophylactic use of supplements, whether or not these two hypotheses turn out to be correct.
>
> The present data suggest that users who have been on supplements for more than five years are at increased risk of breast cancer. The net effect on years of life might still be positive as longer term use may be much less attractive for precisely that reason; women are concerned by such risks and might be inclined to stop before five years.'

However, many workers in this field would suggest that 9-10 years is the accepted duration of safe use before there is increased risk of breast cancer.

The problems of HRT in relation to breast cancer have been reviewed by Howell and his team, working at the Christie Hospital, Manchester[19]. He is cautious about the conclusions of the Nurses' Health Study and argues that an overview of the analyses dealing with 10 or more years' use in the general population show only 30% increased risk after 10 years. There is no evidence of increased **mortality** from breast cancer in women on HRT.

Only one small, randomised, controlled study[20] of 84 women on continuous HRT and 84 on placebo has been published and after 22 years of follow-up no cancer occurred in HRT users, whereas seven controls developed breast cancer. It is hoped that large, randomised studies being launched by the MRC and American NIH will provide answers to these questions.

Family history

Women with a family history of breast cancer are known to be at increased risk. If a woman has one or two first-degree relatives with breast cancer below the age of 60, her risk may be increased by a factor of two or more until she herself reaches 60. Her risk then declines to that of women in the general population.

Howell has provided a meta-analyses of the risk of taking HRT in women with a positive family history (*Table 3.3*).

Table 3.3   Overviews of relative risks of E/HRT use in women with a family history of breast cancer

Authors	Family history	No family history
Armstrong 1988	1.25 (0.83-1.88)	1.01 (0.95-1.06)
* Steinberg *et al* 1991	3.4 (2.0-6.0)	1.5 (1.2-1.7)
Blair 1994	1.2 (0.7-2.2)	1.3 (1.1-1.5)
Steinberg and Smith 1994	1.57 (1.14-2.15)	1.26 (1.11-1.47)
Colditz *et al* 1992	1.07 (0.73-1.56)	1.11 (0.94-1.31)

Howell asked the authors* for further analysis of the 'outlier' paper by Steinberg and the following excerpt is taken from his paper in the *Journal of the British Menopause Society*[19]:

'In her original paper Steinberg reported that the relative risks in patients with a family history were 3.4 (confidence intervals 2.6-6.0) whereas women without a family history, in her analysis, had a relative risk of 1.5 (confidence intervals of 1.2-1.7). We were concerned about the validity of this very large increase in risk and asked Valerie Blair of Manchester Children's Tumour Registry to re-analyse the data. Blair (1994) found no increase in risk in women with a family history when she re-analysed the studies used by Steinberg. Steinberg and Smith (1994) agreed with the re-analysis. They did a further analysis adding two other studies and their recalculated risks are shown in [Table 3.3]. The recalculation showed there was no significant difference between risk of HRT use in women with and without a family history.'

However, the absolute risk remains high if there is a positive family history. Howell then went on to analyse the data relating to women who had biopsy of the breast which showed proliferative breast disease, and also a family history. Although this group had a very high risk of breast cancer (up to 11-fold), when HRT users were compared with non-users the analysis showed reduction of breast cancer in the HRT-related group. **A history of benign breast disease does not contraindicate the use of HRT**. Women with hormonal factors, such as an early menarche, have been studied and there are conflicting reports on the effect of the HRT in this group.

Breast cancer which occurs in women on HRT

The Swedish study found that women who took HRT within a year of cancer diagnosis had greater survival compared to non-users. However, this may have been due to better supervision and earlier grade of tumours.

Can women with breast cancer take HRT?

Traditionally it has been the practice to stop HRT if a patient is diagnosed as suffering from breast cancer. It is also standard advice to regard breast cancer as a contraindication to starting therapy. Small non-randomised studies comparing breast cancer patients using HRT with non-users have not found detrimental effects.

HRT in women taking tamoxifen

These women suffer side-effects of flushes and sweats and may benefit from HRT. The only way to progress is via well-designed trials. A feasibility trial of estrogen replacement therapy (ERT) for women immediately after surgery for breast cancer is under way at the Royal Marsden Hospital in which women are randomised to ERT or no ERT and stratified to adjuvant tamoxifen usage. The UKCC are planning a trial in advanced breast cancer where patients starting tamoxifen will be randomised to receive oestradiol valerate 1 mg daily and medroxyprogesterone acetate (MPA) 10 mg daily versus tamoxifen plus placebo. The aim of the study is to determine whether HRT affects the response rate and the quality of life of patients.

Family history clinics

Referral is usually made through the general practitioner. Under the age of 50, screening should start at an age 10 years younger than the age at which breast cancer was diagnosed in the youngest first-degree relative.

Effect of oestrogen on endometrium

Long-term risks of oestrogen therapy include increased incidence of endometrial cancer. However, this is totally eliminated by sufficient use of progestogen supplements. There is some evidence that endometrial carcinoma is *less* common in users of cyclical oestrogen/ progestogen than in the general population of peri- and post-menopausal women who are not taking hormones.

Stimulation of the endometrium continues for several years after a woman has used unopposed oestrogen or implants. It is important to screen new patients who request HRT and may have previously been given oestrogen without progestogen. Prescription of supplemented HRT to these patients can result in irregular or heavy bleeding due to pre-existing endometrial hyperplasia which may be atypical. Vaginal ultrasound and/or endometrial biopsy are useful investigations. Accurate diagnosis is essential and the management may include cyclical progestogens, repeated curettage or even hysterectomy. This will affect the choice of HRT prescription. Women who have had a hysterectomy for endometrial carcinoma are sometimes advised to avoid oestrogen. Progestogens such as norethisterone are safe and protect against loss of bone density and menopausal symptoms.

Side-effects of progestogens

'Premenstrual' depression, bloating, weight gain and headaches are common complaints in women using cyclical progestogens. It is worth considering changing their HRT prescription to one containing a less androgenic progestogen, such as dydrogesterone or MPA (see Chapter 4).

Dislike of bleeding

Post-menopausal women dislike bleeding and this is a common reason for refusing to consider HRT. *Livial* (tibolone) is partly androgenic, progestogenic and oestrogenic and does not stimulate the endometrium. It is a useful alternative in women who are at least a year past the menopause. Use in younger women may cause irregular spotting. Most women feel well on this preparation and it has been shown to protect against osteoporosis, but there is no evidence that it is cardioprotective. Continuous oestrogen/progestogen is now available in calendar packs and is popular with older women. It may cause unacceptable irregular bleeds if used during the perimenopause.

Considerable research has been carried out on the endometrial safety of these preparations.

Weight gain

Weight gain is commonly mentioned as the reason for not taking HRT. Several controlled studies have not found overall gain in mean weight in oestrogen users, but individual women may put on several kilograms. This may be partly due to retention of sodium/water and is sometimes treated with diuretics. A woman may gain weight on one preparation and not on another. It is worth experimenting with a change of preparation for an individual patient.

Anxiety

There is no doubt that the most important reason for women not to consider HRT is their anxiety about a possible raised risk of cancer. Our own survey of compliance and non-compliance among long-term users showed this and it was also evident in the Oxford survey (see Chapter 6). Many women need more information and it is a sad fact that their chief source of information is often not the family doctor but advice from friends, television programmes, newspapers and women's magazines. They are at the mercy of the media and may build up an unbalanced picture of the risks of therapy. A feeling that they would prefer to live their lives using only 'natural' methods, such as exercise and diet, is the background for many women's cautious approach to HRT. I have some sympathy for this view and would prefer to regard hormone therapy as only one of a series of preventive health measures in a spectrum which includes the use of sunlight, non-smoking, dietary calcium, weight-bearing and aerobic exercise, and a low-fat diet. However, HRT is a necessary option for some high-risk patients with osteoporosis, heart disease or early menopause, and all women should receive balanced and accurate information which is best given around the time of the menopause.

Summary

Use of HRT for between 10 and 20 years increases the risk of developing breast cancer. It does not increase the risk of dying from it. Use for less than five years does not increase breast cancer risk. Women should discuss with their doctor the balance of risks and benefits and make an appropriate decision for their individual needs. Women with a first-degree relative with premenopausal breast cancer should be screened if possible 10 years before the age of diagnosis in their relative.

Useful advice and leaflets are issued by centres such as the Royal Marsden Hospital. The following is an excerpt from their leaflet for general practitioners.

'What to prescribe

We recommend a low-dose combined oestrogen (0.625 mg of conjugated equine oestrogen) and progestogen HRT with tamoxifen.

A combined preparation is recommended both to protect the uterus and because of the theoretical risk of an unopposed oestrogen environment on the breast. The action of tamoxifen is complex and it is not simply an oestrogen antagonist. It is known to decrease the risk of developing breast cancer thus it would seem logical to add it to HRT if patients are not already on it.

Although we do condone the pragmatic use of HRT in women who have had breast cancer there is clearly a need to closely study its risks and benefits in these women. To this end a national trial is being devised which we hope will elucidate the nature and extent of these risks and benefits so that in the future we can offer our patients a more informed choice.

It should be stressed that any patient who has had breast cancer and wishes to use hormone replacement therapy should be carefully monitored by a specialist centre.'

References

1. Chapuy MC, Arlot ME, Delmas PD et al. Effect of calcium and cholecalciferol treatment for three years on hip fractures in elderly women. Br Med J 1994; **308**: 1081-2.

2. Compston JE. HRT and osteoporosis. Br Med Bull 1992: **48** (2): 309-44.

3. DoH. Report of Advisory Group on Osteoporosis. London: HMSO, November 1994.

4. Bush et al. The incidence of death caused by heart disease. Circulation 1987; **75** (6): 1102-9.

5. Stampfer MJ, Colditz GA, Willett WC et al. Post-menopausal oestrogen therapy and coronary heart disease: Ten year follow-up from the Nurses' Health Study. N Engl J Med 1991; **325**: 756-62.

6. Bush TL, Barrett-Connor E, Cowan LD et al. Cardiovascular mortality and non-contraceptive use of estogen in women: results from the Lipid Research Clinics Program Follow-up Study. Circulation 1987; **6**: 1102-9.

7. Volterrani M, Rosano G, Coats A *et al.* Estrogen acutely increases peripheral blood flow in post menopausal women. *Am J Med* 1995; **99**: 119-22.

8. Gangar KF, Vyas S, Whitehead M *et al.* Pulsatility index in carotid artery in relation to transdermal oestradiol and time since menopause. *Lancet* 1991; **338**: 839-42.

9. Mattson LA, Samsioe G, Schoultz B Von *et al.* Transdermally administered estradiol combined with oral medroxyprogesterone acetate: the effects on lipo-protein metabolism in post menopausal women. *Br J Obstet Gynecol* 1993; **100**: 450-3.

10. The Coronary Drug Project. Findings leading to discontinuation of the 2.5 mg/day estrogen group. The Coronary Drug Project Research Group. *JAMA* 1973; **336**(6): 652-7.

11. Boston Collaborative Drug Surveillance Program. Surgically confirmed gallbladder disease, venous thromboembolism, and breast tumours in relation to post-menopausal estrogen therapy. *New Eng J Med* 1974; **290**: 15-9.

12. Young RL, Goepfert AR, Goldzieher HW. Estrogen replacement therapy is not conducive of venous thromboembolism. *Maturitas* 1991; **13**: 189-92.

13. Coope J, Thomson J. Effects of "natural oestrogens" on menopausal symptoms and blood clotting. *Br Med J* 1975; **4**: 139-43.

14. Daly E, Vessey MP, Hawkins MM *et al.* Risk of venous thromboembolism in users of hormone replacement therapy. *Lancet* 1996; **348**: 977-80.

15. Davey DA. The menopause and climacteric. In: *Dewhurst's textbook of obstetrics & gynaecology for postgraduates.* Oxford: Blackwell, 1986.

16. McPherson K. Breast cancer and hormonal supplements in post-menopausal women. *Br Med J* 1995; **311**: 699-700.

17. Bergkvist L, Adami H-O, Persson I *et al.* The risk of breast cancer after estrogen and estrogen-progestin replacement. *New Eng J Med* 1989; **321**: 294-7.

18. Colditz GA, Hankinson SE, Hunter DJ. The use of estrogens and progestins and the risk of breast cancer in post-menopausal women. *New Eng J Med* 1995; **332**: 1589-93.

19. Howell A, Baildam A, Bundred N *et al.* Should I taken HRT Doctor? Hormone replacement therapy in women at increased risk of breast cancer and in survivors of the disease. *J Brit Men Soc.* 1995 Vol 1 (2).

20. Nachtigall MJ, Smillen SW, Nachtigall RD *et al.* Incidence of breast cancer in a 22 year study of women receiving estrogen-progestin replacement therapy. *Obstet Gyneacol* 1992; **80**: 827-30.

CHAPTER **FOUR**

Developing a drug-based strategy of management

Prescribing hormone therapy

E ach general practice team needs to discuss how it is going to manage the menopause and to formulate a policy on prescribing. Even those doctors who regard the menopause as a natural event which does not need to be treated will be required to consider the pros and cons of hormone therapy as patients may ask for it.

There is plenty of evidence that oestrogen therapy is effective in preventing osteoporosis if it is taken for five to 10 years after the menopause, and also that oestrogen reduces the risk of ischaemic heart disease (illness and death) in current users. There is also an increased incidence of about 30% in the risk of developing breast cancer (but not of dying from it) in women who take HRT for over 10 years. The consensus is that oestrogen is a valuable treatment which should be carefully monitored, and thus meticulous assessment and screening are necessary to decide which patients should take it. Education of patients is a *sine qua non* and all women need this even if they decide against hormone therapy. A dedicated menopause clinic is an alternative to *ad hoc* surgery consultations and patients prefer this arrangement. Two hours work each week by a doctor and a nurse is usually sufficient for a surgery with a practice list of 10,000 patients, plus monthly educational sessions for middle-aged women which may involve a counsellor, physiotherapist or dietitian.

Principles of prescription

In women with a uterus, progestogen should be used to eliminate the risk of endometrial cancer. Sequential preparations use progestogen for 10-14 days each month (recently one has been developed using it for 14 days in three months) and the woman usually bleeds after withdrawal of progestogen. About 10% of users have atrophy of the endometrium and never bleed, but this is not dangerous as long as sufficient progestogen has been taken. In the first three months of therapy it is common to experience irregular bleeding as the patient's own endogenous oestrogen produces endometrial stimulation in addition to that provided by the drug. After this time the patient should bleed regularly in a cyclic rhythm and heavy or irregular bleeds need investigation. Continuous oestrogen/progestogen has been developed for women who are at least a year past menopause and irregular spotting is common in the first few months, disappearing altogether in 80% of patients after a year.

Women who have had a hysterectomy should take oestrogen without progestogen. There is no satisfactory evidence that progestogen protects against breast cancer.

Safe doses of progestogen

* Continuous: Norethisterone 1 mg daily

Medroxyprogesterone acetate 5 mg daily

Dydrogesterone 10 mg - 20 mg daily

* Cyclic: Norethisterone 1 mg 10 - 12 days/28

Levonorgestrel 75 - 250 µg 12/28

Norgestrel 150 µg 12/28

Medroxyprogesterone acetate 10 mg 14/28

Medroxyprogesterone acetate 20 mg 14/91

Dydrogesterone 10 mg - 20 mg 14/28

Many women experience progestogenic side-effects, such as bloating, depression, headaches and appetite increase, which are similar to the symptoms of premenstrual syndrome before the menopause. Because of this it is advisable to reduce the dose of progestogen to the lowest which can produce a satisfactory secretory change in the endometrium. One cannot be sure that a patient starting HRT for the first time does not have a pre-existing uterine problem, such as a polyp or atypical hyperplasia, which may only come to light when she starts taking oestrogen. Some women have heavy or irregular bleeding in spite of adequate dosage with progestogen and they need to be investigated. Initial examination of the pelvis and enquiry about bleeding are essential before starting therapy and, if in doubt, vaginal ultrasound is a useful screening test:

Endometrial double thickness < 4 mm	normal post-menopausal
Endometrial double thickness > 8 mm	possibly abnormal

Progestogen only

Norethisterone 5-15 mg daily can be prescribed for women with a history of atypical hyperplasia or endometrial carcinoma, or other contraindication to oestrogen. It is effective against flushes and protects bone density. We have no epidemiological evidence as to the effect on heart disease, but blood lipoprotein assay shows adverse change in HDL/LDL in women taking androgenic progestogens.

Oestrogen dose

It is important to use a preparation which provides adequate plasma oestrogen levels to prevent flushes and also protects against loss of bone density (Table 4.1). *Figure 4.1* shows the plasma level achieved by commonly-used preparations.

Table 4.1   **Doses which are regarded as sufficient to conserve bone**

Bone conserving steroids	Minimum daily doses in common use	
Conjugated equine oestrogens	0.625 mg*	
Piperazine oestrone sulphate	1.5 mg	
Oestradiol 17-beta (oral)	2.0 mg	equally effective
Oestradiol 17-beta (gel)	5 g (= 2 mg)	with progestogen
Oestradiol 17-beta (implant)	50 mg (six monthly)	
Oestradiol 17-beta (transdermal)	50 µg daily	
Norethisterone	5-15 mg daily	
Tibolone	2.5 mg (awaits formal product licence for prevention of osteoporosis)	

*These doses are used for five years post-menopause in healthy women. Lower doses may suffice for older women; younger women with premature menopause may require higher doses.

Figure 4.1 Oestradiol plasma levels and HRT.

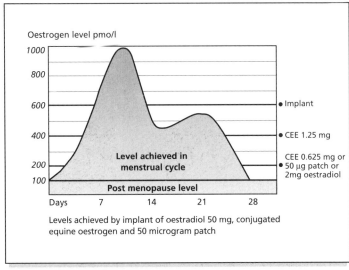

Reproduced with permission from the RCGP.

Different ways of administering oestrogen

When oestrogen is taken by mouth it is absorbed from the gut and passes to the liver in the portal system. Here a considerable part is conjugated and excreted. In passing through the liver (first-pass effect) oestrogen causes increased production of liver proteins, particularly the sex hormone-binding globulin (SHBG), cortisol-binding globulin and thyroxine-binding globulin. SHBG binds selectively to testosterone and this increases the clinical effect of oestrogen (see Figures 1.11 and 1.12).

The increase in cortisol-binding globulin may affect the clinical control of asthma in corticosteroid-dependent patients and they need to be supervised carefully. Thyroid function tests are sometimes affected by the increase in thyroid hormone-binding globulin (THBG). The oestrogen effect on liver function is beneficial in that it improves the lipid pattern, causing increased HDL, lower LDL and reduced cholesterol levels.

Each ingested oestrogen tablet causes a quick temporary rise in plasma oestrogen levels (the bolus effect) followed by a fall. Because such a

67

large portion of oral oestrogen is destroyed quickly, the dose of oral preparations is much higher than that of transdermal preparations. Patches are applied every three to four days and achieve a more even plateau of plasma oestrogen. The high-dose vaginal preparations, such as pessaries, have the same problem as oestrogen tablets, with rapid rise and fall of plasma oestrogen level *(Figure 4.2)*.

Figure 4.2   Short-term variation in oestradiol concentrations with oral, patch and implant therapy.

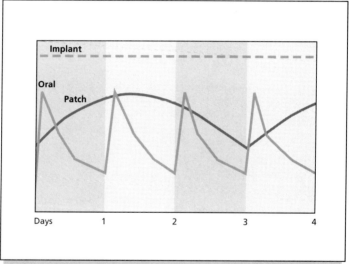

Reproduced with permission from the RCGP.

Women with migraine may be helped by oestrogen patches or implant rather than tablets or vaginal preparations. Oestrogen pessaries can produce a sudden change in oestrogen level - it is the change in level which may produce symptoms of flushing or headaches *(Figure 4.3)*.

Women wishing to stop implant treatment are appropriately treated with patches (sometimes double or treble the 50 µg dose is necessary in young women and this can gradually be reduced). Oestrogen gel is also very effective. Both these preparations use the same drug, oestradiol, which is administered systemically, avoiding the gastrointestinal tract and subsequent reduction of levels via the portal system and liver.

Figure 4.3 Plasma levels (mean ± SEM) of oestradiol after vaginal O and oral ● administration of oestradiol[1].

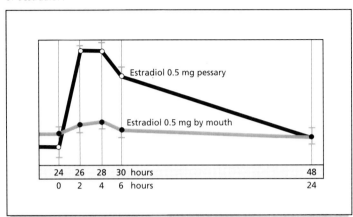

Estradiol 0.5 mg pessary

Estradiol 0.5 mg by mouth

24	26	28	30 hours	48
0	2	4	6 hours	24

Reproduced with the permission of the authors and publishers from: Nahoul K, Denhennin L, Jondet M, Roger M. Profiles of plasma estrogens, progesterone and their metabolites after oral or vaginal administration of estradiol or progesterone Maturitas 1933; 16: 185-202.

New forms of hormone therapy

Continuous oestrogen/progestogen

When women are past the menopause they do not wish to bleed again. The possibility of post-menopausal bleeding is one of the chief reasons for older women deciding against hormone therapy. A great deal of research has gone into the development of bleed-free HRT for older women and the first two preparations below have recently entered the British pharmacopoeia.

Kliofem

Kliofem is continuous oestradiol (2 mg) and norethisterone (1 mg) supplied together in a single yellow tablet. It is taken once daily without a break, supplied in a circular calendar pack. It is only suitable for women who are more than one year post-menopause. Younger women tend to bleed irregularly and spotting can occur in older women during the first few months of treatment. After a year, nearly all users experience amenorrhoea and endometrial atrophy (*Figures 4.4 and 4.5*). If unacceptable bleeding occurs, treatment should stop; if it continues over three weeks, endometrial biopsy should be arranged.

It is highly effective against flushes, vaginal changes and bone loss. Cholesterol and LDL cholesterol decrease by 20% with long-term use. Only one prescription charge is levied. *Kliofem* has been used for over 10 years in Scandinavia.

Figure 4.4 Distribution of patients with at least one episode of bleeding during different months of treatment with *Kliofem*.

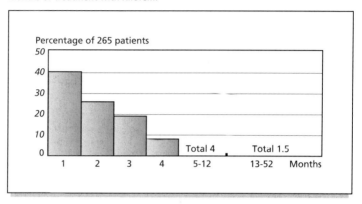

Figure 4.5 Endometrium during different phases of treatment with *Kliofem*.

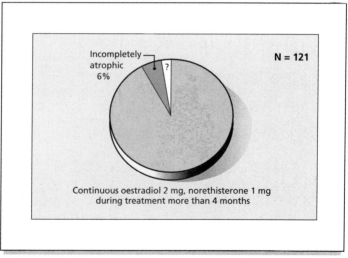

Reproduced with permission from the copyright owner from: Staland B. Continuous treatment with a combination of estrogen and gestagen - a way of avoiding endometrial stimulation. Acta Obstet Gynecol Scan Suppl 1985; 130: 29-35.

Climesse

This is also a once-daily tablet containing 2 mg of oestradiol and 0.7 mg of norethisterone providing bleed-free HRT.

Premique

This is a combination of conjugated oestrogen 0.625 mg with medroxyprogesterone acetate (MPA) 5 mg taken continuously by women at least a year post-menopause.

A controlled study of 1,724 post-menopausal women in the US and Europe showed that about 50% developed complete amenorrhoea after six months' use. Among the patients with valid biopsy data none of the patients receiving this preparation had endometrial hyperplasia.

Matrix patches

Estraderm MX is an example of a matrix patch (applied directly to the skin with alcohol-free adhesive). It is available in three strengths supplying 25 µg, 50 µg or 100 µg of oestradiol per 24 hours depending on patient response. It relieves symptoms such as hot flushes as well as offering longer-term effects in preserving bone density and a beneficial effect on lipids. There is a lower incidence of skin irritation than occurs with alcohol reservoir patches. Another example of a matrix patch is *Fematrix*, which is supplied at a strength of 80 µg oestradiol per 24 hours.

Sequential preparations

Femoston is sequential HRT in tablet form, comprising oestradiol 2 mg for 14 days and oestradiol 2 mg plus progestogen for 14 days.

It is available now in two strengths:

Femoston 2/10

- *Oestradiol (Zumenon) 2 mg 14 days*

- *Oestradiol (Zumenon) 2 mg + 10 mg dydrogesterone (Duphaston) 14 days*

and

Femoston 2/20

- *Oestradiol (Zumenon) 2 mg 14 days*

- *Oestradiol (Zumenon) 2 mg + 20 mg dydrogesterone (Duphaston) 14 days*

A third strength is now available: *Femoston* 1/10.

The reason for yet another sequential HRT is that dydrogesterone is lipid-friendly and does not have the adverse effects on lipids seen with norgestrel or norethisterone. Also, some patients tolerate it better than the androgenic progestogens. A single prescription charge is levied as the oestrogen/progestogen are together in a single tablet.

14 days' rather than 12 days' progestogen is probably necessary because dydrogesterone is relatively 'weaker' than norethisterone in its effect on the endometrium.

Three-monthly bleed

Tridestra contains oestradiol valerate 2 mg given daily for 70 days followed by 14 tablets of estradiol 2 mg combined with medroxyprogesterone acetate 20 mg, followed by seven days' placebo tablets. Bleeding occurs on withdrawal of progestogen during the placebo week. In effect, the patient bleeds every three months. This solves many problems, particularly that of the perimenopausal patient who is going on holiday and wishes to postpone her period. Surprisingly, few women suffered from irregular bleeding when this preparation was studied in 227 women in Finland. These women were post-menopausal and it is noteworthy that the investigators found a higher incidence of heavy unscheduled bleeding in women who had been post-menopausal for less than three months.

Oestrogen gel

Oestrogen gel has been used for many years in France and Spain. Data on absorption are satisfactory and show that it produces effective levels in serum, but there are no available data on prevention of osteoporosis or heart disease.

100 g *Oestrogel* contains 60 mg oestradiol and it is packaged in a canister which dispenses 1.25 mg containing 0.75 mg oestradiol. Two measures daily are the usual dose, delivering 1.5 mg oestradiol 17-beta. Usually, the preparation is effective against flushes after two to

three weeks; if not, the dose can be increased after a month to four measures daily (3.0 mg 17-beta oestradiol). A paper template is provided to show the area over which the gel is rubbed in; over arms, shoulders or thighs (not near the breasts or vulva).

Patients with a uterus need to take additional progestogen. The dose of oestrogel which is recognised to be effective in preserving bone density is 2.5-5.0 g daily but it has not yet received a UK product licence for prevention of osteoporosis. Patients with implants, suffering from tachyphylaxis or simply wishing to stop implants, can often be helped by changing to oestrogen gel which provides the same drug systemically.

Impregnated ring

Estring is a silicone ring impregnated with oestradiol (55 mm diameter). It can easily be inserted and removed by the patient, using water for lubrication. It delivers 7.5 µg oestradiol/24 hours and it is effective over three months. After an initial surge it does not increase serum levels of oestrogen. It is highly effective in improving vaginal lubrication and cytology, and a controlled trial has shown that it improves urinary symptoms and reduces incidence of recurrent urinary infections in older women. It is a lot less messy than pessaries or cream. It is not, of course, effective in treating hot flushes or preventing osteoporosis.

Latest research

Research has shown that oestrogen prevents bone loss over the age of 70 and indeed at any age past the menopause. The Nurses' Health Study[1], which collected data from 121,000 American women, has shown that current use of HRT in older women gives 40% protection against ischaemic heart disease. It is therefore feasible to use oestrogen for preventive treatment in women who are well past the menopause.

Some women will use HRT for a short time in their 50s and then wish to re-start treatment in their 60s or 70s. Others may wish to defer treatment until they have more information, which should be available in 10 or more years from the American National Institutes of Health and the British Medical Research Council randomised, controlled trial commencing 1996-7.

Some women may be doubtful about HRT, and may decide to enter the MRC randomised trial now being set up through the research framework of general practices. They can be reassured that entering the trial will not be detrimental, as hormone therapy begun at a later age will still be effective *(Figure 4.6)*.

Figure 4.6   Metacarpal mineral in subjects commencing mestranol six weeks (0), three years (3) and six years (6) after hysterectomy and bilateral oophorectomy in a placebo group.

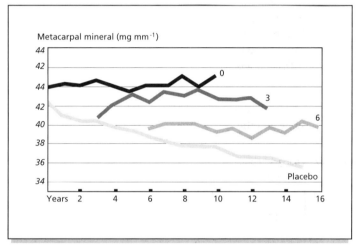

Reproduced with the permission of the author. from: Hart DM. Long-term follow-up of women on HRT. In: HRT and Osteoporosis. JO Drive and JWW Study (ed). London: Springer-Verlag 1990.

For how long should I take HRT?

Women often ask this question. The answer depends on whether she is taking it to:

- alleviate symptoms;

- prevent heart disease or fracture; or

- treat already existing heart disease or osteoporosis.

Symptom control

Menopausal symptoms, such as flushes and insomnia, are improved by HRT and always recur, to some extent, when treatment stops. Many women take therapy for a few months, perhaps up to two years around the time of the menopause in order to alleviate symptoms.

Prevention

The two controlling factors in deciding whether a woman develops osteoporosis are the peak bone mass at menopause and the rate at which she loses bone after the menopause. Primary care doctors have the chance to influence the attainment of satisfactory peak bone mass in patients by trying to prevent young people smoking, encouraging healthy diet and ensuring that antenatal care includes advice on calcium intake, and promoting exercise and the use of local cycle paths and leisure centres.

Hormone therapy is extremely effective in preserving bone density at the level at which the patient starts therapy and protects both the spine and the peripheral skeleton *(Figure 4.7)*.

Figure 4.7   Changes in bone density throughout life.

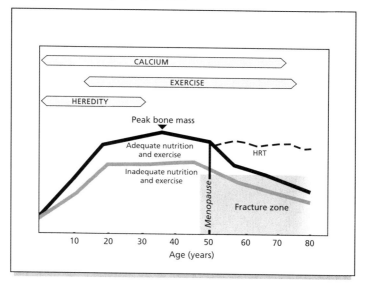

Stopping hormone therapy

Figure 4.8 shows the hot flushes counted per week in two groups of menopausal women. Some were well past the menopause and were trying oestrogen treatment as a possible cure for conditions such as joint pains, vaginal atrophy or fatigue, and had not experienced any flushes for over 10 years. After withdrawal from oestrogen at the crossover to placebo all the women began to suffer from hot flushes, even those who had never experienced them previously. **It is falling levels of oestrogen which precipitate flushes** and it is useful to warn your patients that when they stop therapy they will start having hot flushes. This may go on for several months and recur at any time. They should be informed that flushes are harmless, they do not constitute a disease process of any kind and will eventually disappear.

Figure 4.8 Hot flush count: a six-month crossover trial with conjugated equine oestrogens 1.25 mg^2.

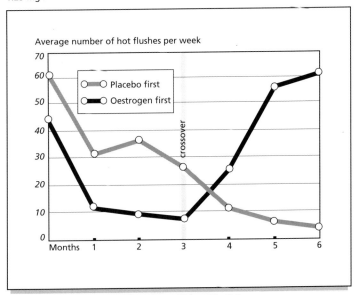

Reproduced with the permission of the authors and Editor of the BMJ.

Many women who stop therapy and experience severe flushes and insomnia may then decide that they have to go back on therapy as they obviously need it. It is these cases that account for so-called oestrogen addiction. Tachyphylaxis on implants is also a problem. Women who are treated with implants may develop high unphysiological levels of circulating oestrogen. When levels fall they experience symptoms, such as flushes and irritability, and may demand a further implant ahead of schedule. It is necessary to measure serum oestradiol levels. If these are high a further implant should be postponed and the patient 'tided over' with oestrogen gel or patches. The decision about whether to continue with long-term therapy should be made on grounds other than symptoms of flushing, and needs careful weighing of the individual risks, benefits and the wishes of the particular patient.

References

1. Stampfer MJ, Colditz GA, Willett WC et al. Postmenopausal oestrogen therapy and coronary heart disease: Ten year follow-up from the Nurses' Health Study. N Engl J Med 1991; **325**.

2. Coope J, Thomson J.M., Poller L. Effects of 'natural oestrogen' replacement therapy on menopausal symptoms and blood clotting. Br Med J 1975; **4**: 139-43.

CHAPTER **FIVE**

Life events and stress around the time of the menopause

Psychological symptoms: how they arise

Evaluation and management

A survey of English and American attitudes to various life events was published in 1976[1]. One hundred and eighty-three English subjects, mostly outpatients and relatives of the psychiatric outpatients at St. George's Hospital, London, and 373 American patients and relatives, were asked to rate various events in terms of the amount of adjustment required to deal with them. *Table 5.1* shows scores which were derived using a scale of 0-20.

Table 5.1 | **Mean scaling scores for 61 events[1]**

Rank in English sample	Event	English Mean	SD	American Mean	SD	Significance*
1	Death of child	19.53	1.91	19.31	1.95	n.s.
2	Death of husband/wife	19.14	2.85	18.83	2.80	n.s.
3	Being sent to gaol	17.76	4.32	17.33	3.62	n.s.
4	Death of close family member	17.65	3.58	16.86	3.76	p<0.05
5	Serious financial difficulties	17.58	3.15	16.53	3.62	p<0.01
6	Husband or wife unfaithful	17.28	4.07	16.80	3.72	n.s.
7	Miscarriage or stillbirth	16.96	4.40	16.05	4.77	n.s.
8	Court appearance for serious offence	16.94	3.78	15.73	4.01	p<0.01
9	Business failure	16.68	3.79	15.99	3.71	n.s.
10	Marital separation due to arguments	16.57	4.20	16.13	4.21	n.s.
11	Unwanted pregnancy	16.48	4.36	15.40	4.93	p<0.05
12	Divorced	16.29	4.93	16.63	4.42	n.s.
13	Fired	15.93	4.80	16.33	4.22	n.s.
14	Death of close friend	15.70	4.06	14.72	4.55	p<0.05
15	Serious illness of family member	15.52	4.21	14.98	4.08	n.s.

Rank in English sample	Event	English Mean	SD	American Mean	SD	Significance*
16	Unemployed for one month	15.43	4.40	14.81	4.39	n.s.
17	Increased arguments with husband/wife	15.01	4.47	12.68	4.73	p<0.001
18	Serious personal physical illness (in hospital or one month off work)	14.67	4.59	14.66	4.18	n.s.
19	Involved in a lawsuit	14.47	4.94	13.21	5.04	p<0.05
20	Fail important exam or course	14.38	4.58	12.86	5.05	p<0.01
21	Losing or being robbed of personally valuable object	14.34	4.69	13.26	4.81	p<0.05
22	Demotion	14.33	4.83	14.75	4.13	n.s.
23	Serious arguments with resident family member (e.g. children)	13.97	4.86	12.63	4.86	p<0.01
24	Begin extramarital affair	13.70	5.53	14.50	4.97	n.s.
25	Taking a large loan (more than half annual salary)	13.64	5.35	12.59	5.31	n.s.
26	Increased arguments with fiancé or boyfriend / girlfriend	13.29	4.81	12.42	4.50	n.s.
27	Break engagement	13.12	5.26	13.01	5.18	n.s.
28	Increased arguments with non-resident family member (e.g.in-laws, relatives)	12.69	4.87	12.01	4.87	n.s.
29	Child marries without approval	12.69	5.68	12.87	5.31	n.s.
30	Increased arguments with boss and co-workers	12.28	5.22	11.67	4.86	n.s.
31	Separation from significant person (e.g. close friend)	12.01	4.80	10.23	4.97	p<0.001
32	Moderate financial difficulties (e.g. increased expenses, debt collectors)	11.90	4.83	10.44	4.93	p<0.01
33	Prepare for important exam	11.41	5.05	10.16	4.89	p<0.05
34	Marital separation not due to arguments	11.33	5.76	9.98	5.44	p<0.05
35	Menopause	11.19	5.62	11.10	5.50	n.s.

Further work by Greene[2] and Cooke[3] in Glasgow demonstrated the importance of life events and the development of symptoms at the menopause. An increase of life events among the general population of climacteric women was mostly due to bereavements, especially the deaths of close relatives.

'The relationship between life events and symptoms was examined in a general population sample of Scottish climacteric women within the framework of the concepts and methods developed in the field of life event research. It was found that at least some of the increase in symptoms at that time of life was due to the occurrence of stressful life events. The relationship was a complex one as different types of life events were associated with symptoms in a differential way. In particular, the occurrence of a bereavement involving a close family member and the consequent loss of social support, were found to be significant factors in provoking physical symptoms but only in the presence of other life stress[2].'

Vulnerability and low self-esteem

Research in Belgium and Switzerland has emphasised the importance of work outside the home in protecting women from menopausal symptoms. This is particularly true for well-educated women who may develop a well-paid and interesting career independently of the family. For other low-paid factory or rural workers the picture is less optimistic. Self-esteem is engendered by a job and a situation in which a woman feels wanted and valued. Brown and Harris have emphasised the importance of self-esteem and also vulnerability factors which make women more likely to develop symptoms and reduce their ability to cope with life *(Figure 5.1)*[4].

'A person's on-going self-esteem - that is, response to loss and disappointment - is mediated by a sense of one's ability to control the world and thus to repair damage, a confidence that in the end alternative sources of value will become available. If self-esteem and feelings of mastery are low before a major loss and disappointment a woman is less likely to be able to imagine herself emerging from her privation. It is this, we believe, that explains the action of the vulnerability factors in bringing about depression in the presence of severe events and major difficulties. They are an odd assortment: loss of mother before eleven, presence at home of three or more children under fourteen, absence of a confiding relationship, particularly with a husband, and lack of a full- or part-time job. (Reversal, of course, will express them as protective factors - not losing a mother before eleven and so on.) We suggest that low self-esteem is the common feature behind all four and it is this that makes sense of them. There are several terms other than self-esteem that could be used almost interchangeably - self-worth, mastery and so on. In the end we chose it because it was a term sometimes used by the women themselves (although they more often talked of lacking confidence). We were particularly interested in a few of the women who took up employment a few weeks after the occurrence of a severe event, none of whom developed depression. One working-class woman who had previously not worked for six years commented that "the money was not much" but it "gave me a great boost" and "greater self-esteem". The relevance for the women of the three vulnerability factors occurring in the present would probably lie in generating a sense of failure and dissatisfaction in meeting their own aspirations about themselves, particularly those concerning being a good mother and wife - this giving them chronically low self-esteem. . . Vulnerability factors play an important role because they limit a woman's ability to develop an optimistic view about controlling the world in order to restore some source of value. Of course, an appraisal of hopelessness is often entirely realistic: the future for many women is bleak. But given a particular loss or disappointment, ongoing low self-esteem will increase the change of general appraisal of hopelessness.'

Figure 5.1   Vulnerability factors.

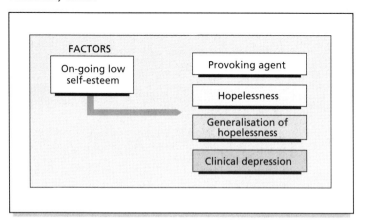

Longitudinal studies of the climacteric

During recent years, four major longitudinal studies of women passing through the menopause have appeared (*Table 5.2*). These have greatly clarified the situation regarding the question of which symptoms are associated with the menopause transition.

Research from North America by McKinlay *et al*[5] addressed the following questions:

• What are the normal menopausal transitions
  and when do they occur?

• What factors affect these transitions?

• What signs and/or symptoms accompany them?

Women randomly selected from annual census lists of those aged 45-55 were contacted by mailed questionnaire and telephone interview of non-responders. In 1982, out of 8,050 responders, 2,570 women were followed through the menopause transition by telephone interviews over five years. The size of the sample and prolonged follow-up enabled the investigators to confirm that the age at natural menopause was 51 years with 1.5 years median difference between smokers and non-smokers. The length of the perimenopausal transition, marked by irregular periods and flushes, was nearly four years. Ten per cent reported abrupt cessation of menses with little irregularity. The peak of hot flushes reported in 50% of women was reached just after the LMP. Four years later only 20% of women complained of flushes. Flushes, sweats and secondary insomnia were the only symptoms consistently associated with menopause. Women found heavy irregular bleeding more troublesome than flushes.

The Manitoba Project[6] sought to examine the possible link between menopause and depression. Since the early 1950s, doctors have assumed such a link and used checklists of symptoms which included depression and irritability despite the lack of supporting evidence. Poor methodology included the use of the Blatt Menopausal Index (not validated by research workers trained in psychological epidemiology). More recently the development of validated scales for measuring depression has assisted more precise measurement of

Table 5.2   Longitudinal studies of menopausal patients

Authors	Country	Population and recruitment	Duration	Symptoms related to menopause and other findings
McKinlay et al[5]	USA	2,570 women aged 45-55 randomly selected from annual census lists Massachusetts. Mailed questionnaires and telephone interviews.	Five years	Flushes in 50% women just after LMP. Insomnia associated with flushes. Irregular bleeding more troublesome than flushes. Smoking accelerated menopause by mean of 1.5 years. Perimenopause lasted nearly four years.
Kaufert et al[6]	Canada	477 women aged 40-59 pre-menopausal or hysterect-omised from mail screen of 2,500 women in Manitoba. Telephone interviews of sub-group of > 45 years old.	Three years	Depression in 25% but impermanent. Not affected by natural menopause. Hysterectomy, family stress and chronic illness associated with depression.
Holte[7]	Norway	200 premenopausal women randomly selected from 1,886 women 45-55 from Oslo Community Register. Yearly personal interview.	Five years	Flushes and sweats + Vaginal dryness + Palpitations + Social dysfunction due to flushes. Depression no change.
Hunter[8]	Britain	36 women out of cross-sectional survey of 850 women aged 47 and over attending ovarian screen clinic London. Postal questionnaire.	Three years	Flushes + Insomnia + Depression + (related to psychosocial factors and negative beliefs)

clinical status. The Manitoba team[6] surveyed by mail 2,500 women aged 40-59 living in Manitoba. A subgroup of responders was followed by six-monthly telephone interviews for three years. In all, 469 women completed five interviews, mean age 48 years. Depression was measured using the Centre for Epidemiological Studies Depression Scale (CES-D). General health, recent family events and stress were recorded. Depression was found to affect 25% of all women interviewed. However, it was relatively short-lived. The Canadian project concluded that depression is common in middle-aged women but is not specifically associated with menopause. They found increased frequency of depression in hysterectomised patients. This does not necessarily imply that hysterectomy causes depression, but previously depressed patients may be more likely to complain of symptoms and to consent to the operation of hysterectomy. Chronic health problems, such as arthritis, were significantly linked with the development of depression.

The Norwegian study[7] randomly selected 200 premenopausal women from a representative sample of 1,886 women aged 45-55 in 1981, whose names were obtained from the Oslo Community Register. Yearly semi-structured interviews lasting three to four hours enquired about work, friends, marriage, family, sexuality and somatic and psychological complaints; gynaecologists and psychologically trained sociologists carried out examinations. Results showed that flushes, sweats, palpitations and vaginal dryness increased at menopause. Psychological complaints were not affected.

Hunter[8] studied a sample of 56 premenopausal women from a cross-sectional survey of 850 women in South-East England. Vasomotor symptoms, insomnia and depressed mood increased during the perimenopause and post-menopause. Previously existing symptoms, negative beliefs and social problems were the most important factors in triggering depression.

These carefully planned and executed surveys confirmed that the natural menopause is not necessarily associated with psychological symptoms. A sudden fall in oestrogen levels, as in castrated younger women, may be associated with loss of libido and depression.

Menopausal myths

Forgetfulness

Forgetfulness is common at all ages and in both sexes. With no firm evidence to support this view, loss of memory has been labelled a 'menopausal symptom'. It is common for women to approach a medical consultation with the words:

"I'm forgetting everything. Is it the menopause?"

The common causes of forgetfulness are anxiety, which blocks the mental processes, and overloading of the memory by having to remember too many detailed facts (a common syndrome in medical students).

Anxiety

This is, of course, common in women who are approaching the menopause. Minor psychological problems are rife at this time and are made worse by the fear of ageing and loss of reproductive life. The infertile woman dreads the last period which will end her hopes of having a child. The insecure woman, fearful of losing her hold on an unreliable partner, may believe that the menopause will reduce her sexual attractiveness.

In our youth-orientated society, millions are spent annually on cosmetics and various forms of beauty treatment in an effort to hold back the years. Cultures such as communities in Rajasthan offer social 'rewards' to women when they cease to menstruate and the incidence of menopausal symptoms is much lower in these countries than in Western Europe and North America. Japanese women have a word 'Konenki' for menopause which describes the life cycle transition. Middle-aged women have a crucial role to play in looking after the elderly. Hot flushes are uncommon, and distressing symptoms are not linked in the Japanese mind to the lack of menses.

Many social problems, such as the care of ageing parents, shortage of money, children's delinquency and lack of support from the partner, may coincide around the time of menopause. Tiredness and poor memory, which result from overwork and worry, are often medicalised by the woman, her family and her doctor, and classified under the diagnostic label of 'the menopause'. Hormone replacement therapy is then prescribed in the hope that the symptoms will disappear.

It is not surprising that many women stop taking HRT after a few months because they are disappointed that it has not met their expectations.

Counselling about personal problems and the appropriate use of hormone therapy can be offered in the surgery as part of primary care. The following letter appeared in the *Journal of the British Menopause Society*[9].

Physician bias: women do need a choice

'Myra Hunter's letter *(March 1995)* indicates the importance of counselling in the menopause clinic. At our osteoporosis clinic we utilised the skills of a nurse counsellor for four years. Her presence has been invaluable not only for giving women accurate information about HRT, but also for providing them with the opportunity to express their concerns. In addition, women are more inclined to discuss any psychosexual problems they are having. At the clinic women are actively involved in deciding if HRT is right for them. Once treatment is started, the role of the nurse counsellor does not end, but she continues to give advice and support through our telephone helpline. Such a broad role for a nurse counsellor has allowed us to achieve high annual compliance rates for HRT and left more time for medical staff at the clinic to concentrate on the clinical assessment of patients. Be it in primary care or in a specialist clinic, we would certainly advocate the involvement of a trained counsellor to assist in the management of women in whom HRT is a treatment option.'

Do oestrogens help psychological problems?

Sudden loss of ovarian activity occurs in young women whose ovaries are removed and the precipitate fall in circulating oestrogen may result in depression, loss of libido and exhaustion. Appropriate hormone replacement is essential. Implants of oestrogen and testosterone are highly effective and later the patient may be weaned off implants and on to high-dose patches or oral therapy.

For older women who experience menopause at an age when oestrogen levels are declining gradually, the evidence is less clear. Double-blind trials show the powerful effect of placebo in at least 70% of patients. Controlled studies have demonstrated that HRT improves sleep, and this may have a positive effect on psychological symptoms - the 'domino' effect.

Effect on sleep

Thomson and Oswald carried out a double-blind study of oestrogen and placebo in perimenopausal women[10] and found that depression, anxiety and hot flushes responded equally to placebo and oestrogen, but oestrogen treatment produced an objective decrease in the brokenness of sleep in perimenopausal women complaining of insomnia.

Conclusions

Careful assessment of the patient's social and psychological background should be part of the initial screening examination. Diagnosis of clinical depressive illness is crucial to effective management and the Beck Depression Inventory (Appendix II) is useful in assessing the depth of depression and suicidal intent.

The difficulty in measuring the effect of HRT on psychological symptoms does not mean that it should be withheld in these patients. It is an extremely safe preparation and compares favourably with many psychotropic drugs for cost, safety and lack of real addictive properties. If a patient is moderately depressed, it is often helpful to prescribe antidepressant medications in addition to HRT.

References

1. Paykel ES, McGuiness B, Gomez J. An Anglo-American comparison of the scaling of life events. Br J Med Psychol 1976; **49**: 237-47.

2. Greene JG. Bereavement and social support at the climacteric. *Maturitas* 1983; **5**: 115-24.

3. Cooke DJ, Green JG. Types of life events in relation to symptoms at the climacteric. Jr Psychomatic Res. 1981; **25**: 5-11.

4. Brown GW, Harris T. *The social origins of depression: a study of psychiatric disorder in women.* London: Tavistock, 1978.

89

5. McKinlay SM, Brambilla DJ, Posner JG. The normal menopause transition. *Am J Hum Biol.* 1992; **4**: 37-46.

6. Kaufert PA, Gilbert P, Tate R. The Manitoba Project: a re-examination of the link between menopause and depression. *Maturitas* 1992; **14**: 143-55.

7. Holte A. Influence of natural menopause on health complaints: A prospective study of healthy Norwegian women. *Maturitas* 1992; **14**: 127-41.

8. Hunter M. The South-East England longitudinal study of the climacteric and menopause. *Maturitas* 1992; **14**: 117-26.

9. Beynon JH. Correspondence. *J Br Men Soc.* 1995; **1** (2): 28.

10. Thomson J, Oswald I. Effect of oestrogen on the sleep, mood and anxiety of menopausal women. *Br Med J.* 1977; **2**: 1317-9.

CHAPTER **SIX**

Follow-up and monitoring strategy

Shared hospital/GP protocols

H ormone replacement therapy spans a wide variety of specialities, although the work of initial screening, selection of patients and long-term supervision falls on general practice. It is helpful for the local gynaecologist and other specialists who are interested to draw up a protocol in consultation with local general practitioners so that they can agree on criteria for referral, indications for bone densitometry and other issues which need to be clarified.

The following excerpt is taken from an article by Dr Jennifer Wordsworth[1]:

'Shared protocols are becoming commonplace, enabling general practitioners to manage their own patients in accordance with national and local specialists' opinion. The Sheffield Protocol for the Management of the Menopause and Prevention of Osteoporosis and the subsequent Sheffield Area Guidelines for Osteoporosis[2] have been well received by clinicians and have raised the quality of patient care. Whilst these protocols could be used in other areas, it has to be recognised that Sheffield is particularly fortunate in having clinicians in all specialities who are pro-HRT and having the support of widely acclaimed accessible specialist services for the menopause and osteoporosis.

The general format for a protocol can be found in the BMS publication 'The management of the menopause'. Specific local policies of clinical specialities which need to be addressed include:

1. **Gynaecologists (general)**

    There are still many who 'don't believe in HRT'.

    Perceived contraindication, history malignant disease, endometriosis etc.

    Indication for routine endometrial sampling and ultrasound.

    Guidelines for referral, e.g. definition of post-menopausal bleeding, fibroids.

2. **Gynaecologists (specialist hospital and community)**

    Guidelines for referral.

    Availability for training and advice.

3. Physicians with special interest in bone disease

Availability of specialist service and indications for referral.

Availability of and indications for bone densitometry.

4. Breast surgeons and radiotherapists

HRT and future risks, e.g. benign breast disease, family history.

HRT with current or past history breast carcinoma.

5. Haematologists

Perceived contraindications.

Availability of and indications for full thrombotic screen.

Indications for investigation and follow-up.

6. Cardiologists

Perceived contraindications.

Attitude to proactive indications.

7. Radiologists

Availability of and indications for bone densitometry (if no specialist unit).

Mammography in relation to national screening programme.

8. Rheumatologists

Screening for steroid takers.

Proactive rationale for HRT.

9. Physicians

Perceived contraindications and follow-up monitoring in relation to other diseases, e.g. diabetes, migraine.

Discontinuation and recommencement of HRT in thromboembolic episodes.

10. Orthopaedic surgeons

Bone densitometry for none/some/all fractures.

11. Anaesthetists/surgeons

HRT non-cessation prior to surgery.'

A joint protocol drawn up by a gynaecologist, two hospital pharmacists and two general practitioners in the Macclesfield area[3] gives guidelines on the history and examination of patients, counselling and management (see algorithm). Detailed advice on contraindications follows.

GUIDELINES FOR THE USE OF HORMONE REPLACEMENT THERAPY

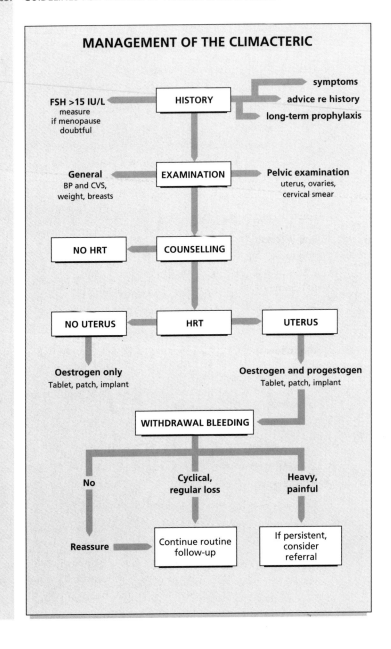

Protocol **Contraindications to HRT**

DEFINITE CONTRAINDICATIONS

Ca breast — At present, should probably be regarded as a contraindication by the non-specialist practitioner. If severe symptoms or a pressing indication, discuss with specialist oncologist/ surgeon.

Ca endometrium — Generally contraindicated, but if disease has been eradicated, may be used (discuss with gynaecologist). Progestogen-only therapy is not contraindicated and may help menopausal symptoms.

POSSIBLE CONTRAINDICATIONS

Many conditions have been wrongly considered as contraindications and in fact are still included in data sheets as a result of inappropriate extrapolation of data derived from the combined oral contraceptive pill. Some of these conditions are considered in the table below.

Characteristic	? Contraindication
Previous thromboembolism	If provoked by prolonged bed rest or surgery, not absolute contraindication. If spontaneous or connected with oral contraceptives or childbirth, the woman's clotting profile should be assessed. This includes antithrombin III, proteins C and S (refer to haematology department). Transdermal oestrogen does not alter coagulation factors.
Ischaemic heart disease	The incidence of fatal MI may be reduced by up to 50% in a woman using HRT.
Cardiac valve disease	Not a contraindication.
Long-term anticoagulation	Not a contraindication.
Hypertension	Treat first. Not a contraindication. Rarely may cause idiosyncratic rise in BP: usually would be manifest at first three-monthly check.
Varicose veins	Not a contraindication.

Protocol		
	Hypercholesterolaemia	Not a contraindication. Oestrogen-only therapy reduces levels, and the oral route is preferable for reduction of cholesterol. Benefits are only marginally opposed by progestogens.
	Hypertriglyceridaemia	Preferably use non-oral route of oestrogen.
	Family history of premenopausal Ca breast in first-degree relative	Family history increases risk of Ca breast, irrespective of exogenous hormone use. Probably not contraindicated for short- or medium-term use (up to five years), but annual breast check/mammography required. Discuss with patient in light of other factors.
	Benign breast disorders	Not a contraindication. Some cystic disease may be reactivated by HRT.
	Uterine fibroids	Not a contraindication. Occasionally increase in size with HRT - do annual vaginal examination.
	Ca ovary	Not a contraindication, but in the rare cases of endometrioid tumours, residual disease may, in theory, be stimulated by oestrogen.
	Abnormal smears/CIN	Not a contraindication.
	Endometriosis	After the menopause, no contraindication to HRT, but disease may rarely be activated. Continuous combined therapy would suppress. Discuss with gynaecologist.
	Malignant melanoma	Probably not a contraindication. Discuss with oncologist.
	Previous other malignant disease	Not a contraindication.
	Gall-bladder disease	Relative contraindication for oral therapy. Hepatic impact may be minimised by transdermal or subcutaneous implant therapy.
	Liver disease	Preferably non-oral route
	Diabetes	Monitor glucose levels carefully. The dose of insulin may need to be adjusted on starting HRT.

Protocol	Epilepsy	Not a contraindication, but anti-epileptic medication may cause liver enzyme induction and accelerate oestrogen clearance. Transdermal therapy is preferable if patient is on phenytoin, phenobarbitone or primidone, and levels should be monitored.
	Migraine	Not a contraindication. HRT will often relieve this, although it may be worsened by progestogen.
	Otosclerosis	May deteriorate in pregnancy, but no evidence that it does with HRT. If in doubt consult ENT specialist.
	Established osteoporosis	HRT can reverse bone loss and increase bone density in established bone disease.
	Smoking	Not a contraindication. Benefits on cardiovascular disease risk are the same and, for this group, of greater importance. Women should be advised that the benefits of HRT will be reduced by smoking.
	Planned surgery	Not a contraindication. *'No information to suggest that HRT should be stopped before surgery.'* (THRIFT consensus group 1992)
	Women over 60	While it is preferable to start HRT at a younger age, research shows that it improves bone density even in women in their 60s and 70s.

Every general practice and hospital trust is unique and has its own problems and merits. These excerpts are merely offered as guidelines so that readers who intend to work with menopausal patients may design their own joint protocols between hospital departments and general practices. Although there are many points at which each party may need to depart from the formal protocol, it is useful to have a framework for co-operation. An increase in meetings and communication between specialists and general practitioners must always work to the advantage of their patients.

Individual practice protocols

When we look at management in each individual practice, it is helpful to have a specialist doctor and nurse who can take a particular interest in the field of the menopause and hormone therapy. Expertise built up over the years is increased by attendance at scientific meetings such as those organised by the British Menopause Society. Again, it is helpful to draw up a formal protocol which serves merely as a basis and checklist for decision making and organisation of premises and personnel.

The following protocol has been recently updated and is derived from our current practice in running a GP menopause clinic over the past seven years. It is not intended as a model to be followed, but as a framework which may be useful to other GP teams to build on when drawing up a protocol for their own practice. Many aspects may need to be modified in the light of a joint protocol with the local hospital (for instance, is the threshold level of FSH for diagnosis of menopause 15, 20 or 30 iu/l?).

The protocol emphasises the use of HRT as preventive medicine in addition to its prescription for short-term symptomatic relief. It does not attempt to persuade women to take hormones but allows them to reach a decision with guidance from the doctor and nurse.

This is the way to improve compliance!

Protocol

FOR DOCTOR/NURSE HRT CLINIC

Aims: To offer screening, prescription, advice and supervision for women wishing to use HRT. HRT is viewed as a preventive strategy against osteoporosis and heart disease.

Manpower: Receptionist/clerk
                     Practice nurse
                     Doctor

Method: Weekly two-hour session at surgery, using two consultation rooms and a reception desk. Patients book on their own responsibility or are referred from one of the partners.

Protocol Appointments: 15 minutes or more depending on problem.

Equipment: Usual gynaecological couch, light etc., wash basin. Computer if generally used in practice. Clinical records.

Clinical protocol

Patients are advised as to the suitability of HRT for them. Accurate diagnosis is essential if complaining of symptoms such as flushes or mood change. Exclude psychiatric illness, social problems, e.g. bereavement, physical illness (i.e. thyroid disease and side-effects of medication).

Contraindications to HRT include:

1. Endometrial or breast cancer (current or past).

2. Present severe thromboembolism, e.g. myocardial infarction or deep vein thrombosis (DVT). Past DVT (especially if due to trauma or obstetrics) or varicose veins are not a contraindication. Previous myocardial infarction is an indication for HRT.

3. Severe liver or kidney disease (prevents efficient metabolism and excretion of oestrogen).

Ethical considerations

1. Patients should be menopausal (periods infrequent or stopped). Although premenopausal women can safely take cyclical oestrogen/progesterone they would often prefer to postpone prescription because of the increased risk of breast cancer with prolonged use. FSH may be used to diagnose menopause in hysterectomised or doubtful cases: >20 iu/l indicates menopause - this depends on your local laboratory (consult them).

2. Patients should be informed about risks and benefits of HRT and decide whether they want it. Has the patient a particular need for HRT (current IHD, early fracture, osteoporosis risk factors etc.)?

   Patients should be informed that breast cancer risks do not escalate under nine years use and should be advised that maximum benefit in osteoporosis prevention is obtained at the menopause when bone loss is most rapid. Current use reduces risk of heart disease.

   Older women: Oestrogen is effective in older women at all ages and many women decide to postpone possible treatment until a few years post-menopause.

Protocol 3. Younger patients who have not yet reached the menopause should be offered contraceptive advice and this may substitute the COC pill for HRT if they do not smoke.

4. Doctor should be aware of other medical problems and treatments, e.g. corticosteroids which increase the risk of osteoporosis.

5. It is useful to have access to bone densitometry which will often help the doubtful patient to decide: "*I will take HRT if bone density is reduced*".

History and examination of patient

Doctor:
Enquire about bleeding: post-menopausal bleeds must be investigated and also bleeding which is irregular, painful or very heavy.

Vaginal examination should be carried out to exclude pelvic masses. If a mass is found it should be investigated before any decision is taken on treatment.

Pelvic ultrasound, endometrial biopsy and/or laparoscopy may be needed.

Nurse:
Breast examination, weight, blood pressure and urine dipstick can be carried out by the nurse (see sample record card).

Mammography:
This is needed for those with a lump in the breast or discharge from the nipple, or family history of breast cancer. It is desirable, but not mandatory, before embarking on long-term therapy. You should insist that the patient accepts a three-yearly mammography screening offered after the age of 50 from the local mammography screening centre. Older women >64 years are not routinely sent for at present. They should be given the telephone number of the centre and encouraged to contact it directly.

After discussion with the patient, history and examination, a decision is made on **whether to offer HRT**. If not, other non-hormonal methods of keeping fit are explained.

Protocol If HRT is decided on, the method is chosen, e.g. patches or tablets (continuous) for hysterectomised patients:

- Patches + progestogen or tablets + progestogen for patients with a uterus. Consider using tibolone after the menopause. Oestrogen gel is now available.

- Local ring or cream or pessaries for vaginal/urethral problems. (Explain that very small doses are needed, otherwise they need progestogen).

Prescription:	by the doctor. Give 3/12 only. Follow-up by appointment with doctor in 3/12, ask about bleeding pattern (may be abnormal in first 2/12 but should regularise after progestogen supplement subsequently). Continuous oestrogen/progestogen at least one year post-menopausal should lead to amenorrhoea after one year. Spotting is common in the early months.
Nurse:	Weight, BP in all initial and follow-up patients. Follow-up yearly or more frequently if there are problems.
Doctor:	Initial prescription 3/12. Follow-up and early assessment in long-term users. Trouble shooting at request of nurse or patient.
	The programme of computerised prescription records can be modified so that all patients on long-term therapy see the doctor every year before a further prescription is issued. Yearly assessment includes breast examination, BP and weight.

Routine questioning of patients:

• *What is the bleeding pattern?*

• *Have you any problems?*

It is better not to question the patient in detail, but you should know the common side-effects of:

oestrogen -	fluid retention, breast enlargement, nausea, headaches (sometimes).
progestogen -	premenstrual syndrome, headache, depression, bloating.

101

Protocol **Sample record card**

FEMALE Surname	Forenames

Address

National Health Service Number   Date of Birth

Date	★	CLINICAL NOTES
		LMP/Symptoms
		Hyst/Ovariectomy
		Contraception
		FH e.g. Osteoporosis, IHD.
		Calcium How many mg daily (see chart)
		Hormones How long used
		UV Sun hours daily
		Smoking Number of cigarettes
		Excercise
		Contrainds
		Alcohol Units/week
		WT Kg } ̶B̶M̶I̶ HT metres }
		BP
		Cholesterol If >7.0 => fasting lipids
		Breast/Mammog
		VE/Smear
		Plan

★ This column has been provided for doctors to enter A,V or C at their discretion FORM FP8

Health education

It is often useful to offer educational sessions to women over the age of 40 to explain the various methods of self-help and the risks and benefits of hormone therapy. At first we organised this in the lunch-hour but, in spite of the enthusiasm of staff and patients, attendance was only 50% of the women who were invited by letter.

Recently an evening session once a month has resulted in large attendances and considerable interest among patients. We have now given up examining patients and simply offer advice. The following protocol is a framework which may be modified considerably to fit in with the preferences of the individual practice.

Protocol

FOR NURSE/DOCTOR WOMEN'S HEALTH CLINIC

A one-off education and screening clinic offered to all women in the practice between the ages of 40 and 60, which educates them about HRT and other preventive strategies against fractures, heart disease and stroke. Also nutrition and family health.

Aims:	Education and screening of all middle-aged women. This clinic feeds the HRT clinic, i.e. it enables women to perceive the uses of HRT and attend the HRT clinic.
Manpower:	Receptionist/clerk Practice nurse Doctor Physiotherapist? Nutritionist?
Method:	Two-hour sessions using two consultation rooms, teaching room, video room.
Appointments:	Patients are identified from age/sex register and contacted in groups. Secretary sends invitation to attend on a specific date or patients attend in response to posters, leaflets or press coverage.

	If you send a letter this should be informative, non-threatening and friendly and explain why we are sending for patients (to educate them and find out lifestyle and health problems).
Equipment:	Blackboard or flip-chart
	Posters showing high calcium diet, healthy heart diet
	Leaflets (e.g. anti-smoking)
	Diet sheets
	Weighing scales, height measure, cholesterol screening, video, TV.

Procedure

1. Patients come to receptionist, then sit in a group for lecture from doctor - s/he gives information on prevention of osteoporosis, risks and benefits of HRT, etc.

2. Patients are each seen by the nurse who completes a data sheet including height, weight, exercise, smoking history, cholesterol (high-risk patients), BP, urine dipstick.

3. Each patient is then seen privately by doctor who completes LMP, hormone use, calcium intake (calculated from chart), examines contraindications to therapy, other health problems, alcohol intake, and demonstrates HRT tablets/patches to patient.

   They make a decision (or postpone one) on whether HRT would be acceptable.

4. Physiotherapist gives monthly exercise class (optional).

   Nutritionist/cook gives monthly cookery class (optional).

5. Videos are used for teaching about osteoporosis.

Prescriptions are only issued after screening breasts and pelvis, and possibly other tests such as mammogram. Patients are followed up in the HRT clinic.

You do not need to hold an education session at the surgery - the local Leisure Centre or Women's Institute Hall is quite appropriate.

Protocol **Typical calcium content of food**

1/3 pint (195 ml) silver top milk..230 mg

1/3 pint (195 ml) semi-skimmed milk ....240 mg

1/3 pint (195 ml) skimmed milk..250 mg

1 oz (28 g) Cheddar or other hard cheese........................220 mg

5 oz (140 g) pot of yoghurt ....270 mg

4 oz (112 g) cottage cheese..60 mg

4 oz (112 g) ice-cream ....157 mg

2 oz (56 g) sardines (including bones) ....220 mg

Two large (60 g) slices white bread....................................60 mg

Two large (60 g) slices wholemeal bread............................14 mg

4 oz (112 g) spring cabbage ....30 mg

4 oz (112 g) broccoli...6 mg

4 oz (112 g) baked beans..45 mg

2 oz (56 g) peanuts...34 mg

2 oz (56 g) dried apricots ....52 mg

Targeting the vulnerable groups

A number of other vulnerable groups would benefit from long-term preventive use of HRT. We assume that it needs to be continued over five years to protect bone density and stopped after 10 years because of the increased risk of breast cancer. The latter point needs to be explained to the patient who may decide that, despite the risk, she would prefer to continue taking oestrogen as in her case the perceived benefit outweighs the risk. It does not apply in cases where the ovaries have been removed.

The vulnerable groups include:

1. Women with early (premenopausal) oophorectomy or ovarian irradiation.

2. Women with hysterectomy before menopause.

3. Long-term corticosteroid users, and

4. Long-term thyroxine users - lead to reduced bone density.

5. Women with family history of osteoporosis, and

6. Women with body mass index <20 - found at women's health clinic.

7. Women with family history of early cardiac death.

8. Women who already have:
   • ischaemic heart disease (IHD)
   • coronary artery bypass graft (CABG)
   • positive coronary angiogram
   • angina

9. Women with two or more raised risks factors for IHD:
   • cholesterol >7.0 mmol/l
   • smoking >15 cigarettes daily
   • BP >160/90 mmHg

Hysterectomy

At the present time, one of the most commonly performed operations in the NHS is hysterectomy. These have increased from 57,000 in 1982 to 67,000 in 1991. The over-35s show a high prevalence of hysterectomy and approximately one in five women will have had a hysterectomy by the age of 55. At the present time, 2.7 million women in the UK have had a hysterectomy. Approximately 210 women aged between 25 and 64 years of age in a five-partner practice of 10,000 would have had hysterectomy and it is estimated that despite long-term use of HRT in hysterectomised women being recognised as cost-effective, less than 30% of these women are receiving HRT. Except for those suffering from breast cancer, most oophorectomised women should receive HRT, but many do not and the majority of those who do start therapy discontinue HRT, for a variety of reasons, after about two-and-a-half years. Identification of these vulnerable patients is now possible because each practice has a list of hysterectomised patients who are excluded from the NHS cervical screening programme.

Oophorectomy

Computerised records can be used to find those whose ovaries were removed before the age of 50. These women, some of whom suffered from an artificial menopause in their 30s, are especially vulnerable to heart disease and osteoporosis. It is important to offer oestrogen therapy from the date of the operation unless there is an over-riding contraindication, such as breast cancer. It should be explained to them that women who are castrated early have substantial reduction in breast cancer risk and it is safe and necessary for them to take oestrogen for 20 years or more. Hysterectomy without removal of the ovaries may precipitate earlier menopause (ovarian failure) because of interference with ovarian blood supply, but recent evidence conflicts with this view and does not show accelerated loss of bone density in these patients. Nevertheless, women who have had a hysterectomy are much more likely to accept HRT because they do not have a problem with bleeding, and it is important to educate them and offer prescription of oestrogen therapy.

Corticosteroid users

Long-term corticosteroid users can be identified from computerised repeat prescription print-outs under headings prednisolone, *Becloforte* etc. You need to set a threshold of corticosteroid use, otherwise you could identify hundreds of low-dose users who may not be at risk. In our practice we set a level of a minimum of inhaled beclomethasone 1 mg daily and any dose of prednisolone or prednisone 5 mg daily and inhaled corticosteroids. This is one area which is eminently suited to general practice/hospital joint protocol or guidelines, particularly as it involves the radiology department in densitometry. When patients are identified as high-dose, long-term corticosteroid users we invite them to attend the surgery to discuss bone density estimation and possible treatment. It is important that the letter should not be too frightening and the final draft of our letter is shown overleaf.

Eighty per cent of those receiving a letter responded, and *Table 6.1* gives details of three of the patients who were identified as being at risk and who are being treated at present.

Table 6.1   Details of three patients at risk of ostoeporosis because of corticosteroid use

Initials	Age	Smoking	Bone density reduction S.D	History	Management
MC	66	Occasional	-2.4	Becl. 3 pred. 5 back pain 2 previous fractures	*Premarin* 0.625 mg *Micronor* 2 daily Calcichew
ML	63	Ex-smoker	-2.8	Parkinsonism Ex-steroids	Offer HRT
EW	34	6 per day	-1.3	Recently widowed asthma Becl. 3 puffs	Calcium Offer HRT

Monitoring therapy

Long-term monitoring of patients on therapy is a task eminently suited to primary care, and the work has become a great deal easier with the advent of computers. This chapter has dealt with the problems of education, screening and monitoring of HRT users. We have also included the monitoring of those dependent on long-term corticosteroids and thyroxine, and those with ischaemic heart disease, and the possibility of treatment of low bone density with HRT. Tibolone and biphosphonates such as etidronate or alendronate are useful options for those who do not wish to take hormones.

In all cases, lifestyle changes are advised which will assist the health of heart and bones:

- Healthy diet
- No smoking
- Exercise
- Moderate exposure to sunlight

Helping patients follow the treatment you prescribe

One of the chief problems with HRT is that patients take it for only a short time. At least five years use is needed to afford measurable protection against fracture and it is current use which protects women against ischaemic heart disease. When we monitored 200 long-term users in our practice we found that hysterectomy was very important in determining whether women took HRT *(Table 6.2)*. Over 50% had had a hysterectomy.

Table 6.2   **Compliance with HRT[a]**

Year	Total no. staying on HRT	No. of users with uterus	No. of hysterectomised users	No. stopping HRT in that year	Compliance*
86/87	88	29	59 (67%)	17	84%
87/88	143	71	72 (50%)	18	89%
88/89	246	125	121 (49%)	21	92%
89/90	284	148	136 (48%)	45	86%
90/91	260	130	130 (50%)	51	84%
*(= No. staying on HRT expressed as a % of no. taking at start of year)					

Reproduced with the permission of the authors and publisher.

Draft letter

Address of

Patient

Here

Dear ....

You may be aware that our practice is very interested in health promotion and we have been looking through your records and find that you are taking long-term corticosteroids (*Becloforte* or prednisolone).

These sometimes have a damaging effect on bone thickness and we now have tests available at [town] on the NHS, which would help us to decide whether you need further treatment to protect you from osteoporosis and fractures.

We would like to invite you to come to the surgery on [date] at [time] when we could discuss, in a confidential interview, whether you need further help. Could you please let us know whether you will be able to keep this appointment. If it is not convenient we can send you another appointment for a later date. If you cannot attend because you are housebound please let us know and we will try to arrange a home visit.

Yours etc.

Another determining factor is the social class and education of the women. The question has been asked: *"is it a particular kind of woman who takes HRT?"* The answer is yes; she is more health-orientated, less likely to smoke, and of a higher social class than the non-user. *Figure 6.1* shows the comparative social class distribution of the women who attended our health education clinic and those who refused the invitation. Clinic attenders were half as likely to smoke, and three times as likely to use HRT as the non-attenders.

When we attempted to find out why women stopped therapy, the most important reasons were problems with bleeding and anxiety about the risks of treatment *(Table 6.3)*.

Figure 6.1   Social class distribution of attenders and non-attenders at the clinic[5].

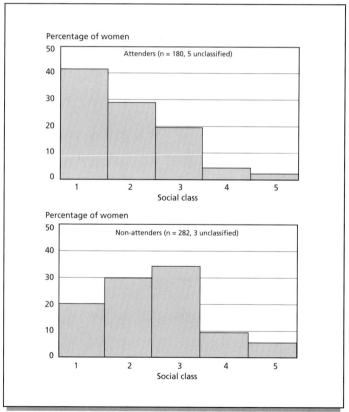

Table 6.3   **Reasons for stopping treatment¹**

Reasons for stopping treatment	Hysterectomised	With uterus
Anxiety about 'unnecessary treatment, cancer or medicalisation of life'	12	13
Bleeding problems, or did not want periods	–	14
Felt unwell	4	6
Breast lumps	3	2
Breast cancer	1	–
Weight gain	3	2
Abdominal pain - oral oestrogen	3	–
Chest pain - oral oestrogen	1	–
? Jaundice	1	–
Knee operation	1	–
Painful veins or thrombosis	1	1
Cystic hyperplasia	–	2
Ovarian cyst	–	1
Migraine or PMS	–	2
Asthma	–	2
Fibroids	–	1
Endometriosis	–	2
Abnormal lipids	–	2
Malignant melanoma	–	1
Fractured spine	–	1
Hyperthyroidism	–	1
Unknown	7	6
Gone away, left list	15	6
TOTAL	**52**	**65**

Reproduced with the permission of the authors and publisher.

A recent survey of 525 users in Oxfordshire showed that[6]:

- The main reason for starting HRT was symptom control.

- Only 49% women obtained their information about HRT from health-care professionals, and thus many did not receive counselling based on their own specific needs.

- Lack of information was more often found in lapsed users.

- Few women know about the cardiovascular benefits of HRT.

- 51% of lapsed users stopped within one year.

- Women stop HRT without consultation with a health-care professional, the most important reasons being unwanted side-effects, the most intolerable being heavy periods which are also the most intolerable perimenopausal symptoms.

Patients need information and education, and easily accessible help and supervision is important in preventing lapses from therapy.

Conclusions

Protocols for use by an individual practice or jointly between specialists and general practitioners are intended for use only as a framework so that doctors can design their own guidelines. Copies of the original Macclesfield Hospital/GP protocol may be obtained from Dr Valerie Ramsden, Bollington Medical Centre, Bollington, Macclesfield, Cheshire or from Mr Stuart Mellor, Macclesfield District General Hospital.

Compliance is an ugly word which seems to imply that there has been manipulation and subjugation. It should not mean this. Helping your patients to stick with the treatment is an essential part of general practice, and adequate and on-going education and communication should enable you to succeed. The patient should always take part in the decision-making process.

References

1. Wordsworth J. Shared-care protocols for the management of the menopause. *British Menopause Society Newsletter*, December 1994, No. 7.

2. Lee S. *The Sheffield protocol for the management of the menopause.*

3. Mellor S, Stirling A, Ramsden V. *Guidelines for the use of hormone replacement therapy: management of the climacteric.* East Cheshire NHS Trust Working Party. Macclesfield District General Hospital, March 1994.

4. Coope J, Marsh J. Can we improve compliance with long-term HRT? *Maturitas* 1992; **15**: 151-8.

5. Coope J, Roberts D. A clinic for the prevention of osteoporosis in general practice. *Br J Gen Pract.* 1990; **40**: 295-9.

6. Hope S, Rees M. Why do British women start and stop hormone replacement therapy? *J. Brit Men Soc* 1995; **1** (2): 26.

CHAPTER **SEVEN**

Personal assessment questionnaires for perimenopausal women

There is a need for questionnaires to assess the wide range of emotional and physical symptoms which are experienced by middle-aged women. Those working in primary care are aware of the diversity of the problems which are labelled 'due to the menopause' and the time-consuming nature of the work that is involved in running a menopause clinic. Although patients can be seen during the course of an ordinary general practice surgery, the 5-10 minute consultation is hardly sufficient for the doctor to assess the possibility that the patient's problem is due to hormonal changes, or may be helped by HRT, perhaps to arrange for FSH or thyroxine estimation, and refer her to the appropriate clinic. We know from Paula Roberts' survey of women patients who attended her clinic in Wigan that patient satisfaction is significantly greater if they are seen at a dedicated clinic, where much more time is available and experienced staff can offer specialised information and expertise.

I still feel that the menopause is a 'general practice area' and that primary care can offer an all-round view which encompasses problems ranging from osteoporosis to marriage breakdown. General practitioners are also aware of the preventive role of HRT and can provide continuity of future supervision that is not always available in hospital clinics. Assessment of women in primary care is helped by having the 'tools' to finish the job, in this case an appropriate and validated questionnaire.

The following is a questionnaire that has been devised by Myra Hunter[1] a psychologist working at Guy's Hospital, London.

Women's Health Questionnaire

Please indicate how you are feeling now, or how you have been feeling in the last few days, by putting a tick in the correct box in answer to each of the following items:

	Yes definitely	Yes sometimes	No not much	No not at all
1 I wake early then sleep badly for the rest of the night.	☐	☐	☐	☐
2 I get very frightened or panic feelings for apparently no reason at all.	☐	☐	☐	☐
3 I feel miserable and sad.	☐	☐	☐	☐
4 I feel anxious when I go out of the house on my own.	☐	☐	☐	☐
5 I have lost interest in things.	☐	☐	☐	☐
6 I get palpitations or a sensation of butterflies' in my stomach or chest.'	☐	☐	☐	☐
7 I still enjoy the things I used to.	☐	☐	☐	☐
8 I feel life is not worth living.	☐	☐	☐	☐
9 I feel tense and wound up.	☐	☐	☐	☐
10 I have a good appetite.	☐	☐	☐	☐
11 I am restless and can't keep still.	☐	☐	☐	☐
12 I am more irritable than usual.	☐	☐	☐	☐
13 I worry about growing old.	☐	☐	☐	☐
14 I have headaches.	☐	☐	☐	☐
15 I feel more tired than usual.	☐	☐	☐	☐
16 I have dizzy spells.	☐	☐	☐	☐
17 My breasts feel tender or uncomfortable.	☐	☐	☐	☐
18 I suffer from backache and/or pains in my limbs.	☐	☐	☐	☐

Women's Health Questionnaire	Yes definitely	Yes sometimes	No not much	No not at all
19 I have hot flushes.	☐	☐	☐	☐
20 I am more clumsy than usual.	☐	☐	☐	☐
21 I feel rather lively and excitable.	☐	☐	☐	☐
22 I have abdominal cramps or discomfort.	☐	☐	☐	☐
23 I feel sick or nauseous.	☐	☐	☐	☐
24 I have lost interest in sexual activity.	☐	☐	☐	☐
25 I have feelings of well-being.	☐	☐	☐	☐
26 I have heavy periods.	☐	☐	☐	☐
27 I suffer from night sweats.	☐	☐	☐	☐
28 My stomach feels bloated.	☐	☐	☐	☐
29 I have difficulty in getting off to sleep.	☐	☐	☐	☐
30 I often notice pins and needles in my hands and feet.	☐	☐	☐	☐
31 I am satisfied with my current sexual relationship (please omit if not sexually active).	☐	☐	☐	☐
32 I feel physically attractive.	☐	☐	☐	☐
33 I have difficulty in concentrating.	☐	☐	☐	☐
34 As a result of vaginal dryness sexual intercourse has become uncomfortable (please omit if not sexually active).	☐	☐	☐	☐
35 I need to pass urine/water more frequently than usual.	☐	☐	☐	☐
36 My memory is poor.	☐	☐	☐	☐

37 Is it very difficult for you to cope with any of the above symptoms?   YES / NO
If so, which ones:

The questionnaire has been specifically developed to measure subjective reports of emotional and physical well-being, and tested extensively in a sample of 682 women, aged 45-65 years, attending a routine screening clinic. This sample was similar in social class distribution and marital status to the population of South-East England. Factor analysis was used to explore the relationship between symptoms. Depressed mood and anxiety formed separate scales, as did sleep problems, menstrual problems, sexual behaviour and vasomotor symptoms. Test and re-test reliability was found to be high when the questionnaire was tested and re-tested in a sample of 48 women. The depressed mood scale was validated against the widely accepted General Health Questionnaire which was published by Goldberg in 1972[2]. The questionnaire is self-administered by the patient. Vaginal dryness is assessed only in relation to sexual intercourse as this is the reason for its presenting as a problem. Sexual interest *(question 24)* is assessed separately from sexual satisfaction *(question 31)*. Depression is assessed by questions 3, 5, 7, 8 10, 12, 15 and 25, some of which are scored in reverse *(7, 10, 25)*. Reversed items provide a useful check on the reliability of answers. The Women's Health Questionnaire detects long-standing problems better than the General Health Questionnaire.

Scoring

Factor scores were derived by summing the symptom scores, recorded as present or absent. ('Yes definitely' and 'Yes sometimes' are scored 1, while 'No not at all' and 'No not much' are scored 0). The factor analysis was performed on a four-point scale, but this was reduced to a binary scale to simplify scoring. For certain items the scoring was reversed as some items were phrased positively and some negatively. The reversed items were 7, 10, 21, 25, 31 and 32. To obtain factor scale scores, the scores on the following items are summed and divided by the number of items in each subscale:

- *Depressed mood:* Items $(3 + 5 + 7 + 8 + 10 + 12 + 25) \div 7$

- *Somatic symptoms:* Items $(14 + 15 + 16 + 18 + 25 + 30 + 35) \div 7$

- *Memory/concentration:* Items $(20 + 33 + 36) \div 3$

- *Vasomotor symptoms:* Items $(19 + 27) \div 2$

- *Anxiety/ fears:* Items $(2 + 4 + 6 + 9) \div 4$

- *Sexual behaviour:* Items $(24 + 31 + 34) \div 3$
- *Sleep problems:* Items $(1 + 11 + 29) \div 3$
- *Menstrual problems:* Items $(17 + 22 + 26 + 28) \div 4$
- *Attractiveness:* Items $(21 + 32) \div 2$

Thus each factor score has a minimum of 0 and a maximum of 1, with 1 reflecting greater symptom experience or more difficulties in a particular area *(Table 7.1)*.

Table 7.1 | 'Normal' scores for women in age bands 45-65 years (means and standard deviations)

General sample			
Age range	45-54	55-65	45-65
Mean age (SD):	49.64	57.66	52.32
	(2.78)	(2.64)	(4.92)
N	474	179	682
WHQ scale scores			
1. Depressed mood:	0.22 (0.22)	0.20 (0.22)	0.22 (0.23)
2. Somatic symptoms:	0.36 (0.25)	0.41 (0.24)	0.39 (0.25)
3. Vasomotor symptoms:	0.44 (0.41)	0.41 (0.43)	0.43 (0.44)
4. Anxiety/fears:	0.35 (0.28)	0.34 (0.29)	0.35 (0.28)
5. Sexual behaviour:	0.28 (0.30)	0.38 (0.32)	0.32 (0.43)
6. Sleep problems:	0.42 (0.35)	0.48 (0.35)	0.45 (0.36)
7. Menstrual symptoms:	0.45 (0.39)	0.26 (0.24)	0.38 (0.29)
8. Memory/concentration:	0.47 (0.36)	0.41 (0.37)	0.47 (0.36)
9. Attractiveness:	0.36 (0.28)	0.40 (0.31)	0.38 (0.29)

When you obtain a score which is significantly above the norm, e.g. depressed mood of 0.66 in a woman of 54, it is helpful to arrange further interview to assess the problem. It may be useful to use further questionnaires, e.g. Beck, Goldberg or Green's Model. It is never a waste of time to call in ancillary workers to help you to make an accurate assessment in a particular patient. You may need help from a psychologist, psychiatrist, social worker, nurse behaviour therapist, bereavement counsellor or relatives. For instance, you may make a provisional diagnosis of 'depression'. You need to know:

• How long has the problem been around?

• Is it getting worse?

• How bad is it?

• Can she work?

• Is she suicidal? *(See Beck Inventory, Appendix II)*

• Are there social circumstances which affect outcome? (e.g. poverty, loss of spouse, job or home, worry about children [call in social worker])

• Anxiety may play a part. See Green's Vulnerability Model *(Chapter 5)* (Illness, poverty, somatic anxiety symptoms). Medical - look up record - use of antidepressants
HRT
tranquillisers
alcohol
cigarettes (number per day)

Quality of life

A recent editorial in the *Lancet*[3] underlines the importance of measuring the quality of life (QoL):

> 'Before a marketing authorisation is delivered, studies of the impact of the treatment on the patient's well-being should be required. One approach . . . is to formally assess quality of life with validated questionnaires.'

Another reason for increasing attention being paid to QoL in medical research is the increased prevalence of chronic diseases with the ageing of society. The outcome in such diseases cannot, by definition, be cured, but must relate to the well-being of patients treated. QoL also influences treatment outcome. Several studies have found that factors such as overall QoL, physical well-being, mood and pain are of prognostic importance for survival of cancer patients. Finally, patients themselves support the need for more attention to QoL, and demand more insight into the concomitants of their disease and its treatment. Breast cancer patients, for example, have expressed their wish for more emphasis on research into QoL issues.

We now know that a patient's self-assessment may differ substantially from the judgement of the doctor or other health-care staff, and some patients' preferences seem to differ from those of others. Many patients accept toxic chemotherapy for the prospect of slight benefit in terms of survival or prolongation of life, contrary to the expectation of medical staff. Moreover, patients' priorities may differ from those of researchers. It has been shown that investigators are currently paying only lip-service to such ideas.

If QoL is so important, and if so many trials organisations are advocating greater use of QoL as outcome measures, why have there been so few publications describing QoL assessments in randomised controlled trials (RCTs)? Undoubtedly, the reason is that large, multicentre RCTs usually take many years to complete; over the next few years we are likely to see a pronounced increase in trials reporting QoL results.

Questionnaires to measure the quality of life

There is a shortage of questionnaires to measure changes in the quality of life which may be due to the menopause itself, or to treatment which is prescribed for menopausal symptoms. Daly[4] and others working at the Department of Public Health and Primary Care at the University of Oxford have devised two different methods of measuring the quality of life in perimenopausal women. The first method used a rating scale. Patients were given a brief non-technical description of typical mild and severe menopausal symptoms and were shown a numerical scale marked 0 to 10 with end-points of 'death' and 'normal health'. The patients were asked to pick points on the scale which represented the quality of life in women experiencing these symptoms. Patients were drawn from women aged 45 to 60, 32 of whom were attending a specialist menopause clinic and 31 from two general practices in Oxford.

The second method, entitled the 'time trade-off method', involved offering a woman two alternatives - a number of years (x) lived at reduced health (defined by the questioner) or fewer years (y) with normal health. Time y was varied until the subject has no preference, and at this point the utility value of life in the state of reduced health is assigned the value of y/x. Subjects were then asked the same question assuming that menopausal symptoms are causing the reduced health state. For example: which would you prefer, 10 years with hot flushes or [ ] years of normal health? This method was tested on the same sample of 63 women, mean age 52.1 years, which consisted of 21 never-users of HRT, 17 HRT users who had experienced mild symptoms, and 25 users who had experienced severe symptoms.

Figure 7.1 Comparison of QoL measurements obtained by different methods ('rating scale' and 'time trade-off').

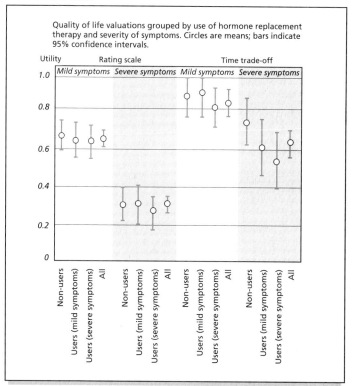

When the 'utility' or 'rating scale' method was used, women's perception was that quality of life was very much reduced by menopausal symptoms. The 'time trade-off method' produced substantially different values and women had no preference for five years of mild symptoms over 4.25 normal years, or five years of severe symptoms over 3.2 years in normal health. HRT users were asked to rate their quality of life before and during treatment, and quality of life ratings significantly increased especially in those women who had experienced severe symptoms.

In the 'time trade-off' method women were unwilling to consider any shortening of the length of life in return for alleviation of menopausal symptoms. This is not surprising as many women do not perceive the menopause as life-threatening or extremely painful (e.g. as compared with terminal cancer pain or biliary colic), and many women lead lives orientated towards altruistic care of others - reasons given included "my handicapped son needs me to care for him". It is interesting to compare the comments with those of Japanese women (see Chapter 5, p.87) who do not complain of menopausal symptoms as their lives are family- rather than self-orientated.

The overall conclusions of this study are that the menopause causes deterioration in the quality of life and that hormone therapy can produce a considerable improvement. Assessment of the cost-effectiveness of HRT needs to include measurement of the quality of life, and this has particular relevance to research protocols in this area (see Appendix I).

The Beck Inventory for measuring depression

This is a sensitive tool which can be used in general practice[5]. It gives an estimate of the depth of depression - whether a patient is slightly sad, down-hearted or suffering from a depressive illness. It may be self-administered by the patient, but I have found it helpful to sit with patients, particularly those who are less used to filling in forms, to explain some of the terms. Repeated use is extremely accurate in demonstrating whether a patient is improving or getting worse. It reflects recent mood. Questions F and I indicate suicidal intent and a high score would suggest the need for early referral to a psychiatrist.

The authors validated the questionnaire by in-depth interviews by four experienced psychiatrists who saw 226 psychiatric patients before or after administering the questionnaire. Replication was carried out in a further group of 183 patients. Highly significant correlations occurred between the two methods of assessment (see Appendix II, p.163).

Our practice has used this questionnaire extensively during a research study to assess the effect of oestrogen on depression and found it a sensitive indicator of recent change in depressive illness. Although depression is not a symptom of menopause, and is not usually due to hormonal changes, there is a high incidence of depression in middle-aged women, often due to social and economic factors. It is not uncommon for a woman to attend a clinic and request hormone treatment because she is 'tired, unable to think properly, sex life is poor, unable to sleep' etc. It is vital to offer proper assessment and diagnosis, and the Beck questionnaire can be very useful. Treatment may be offered in a variety of areas such as antidepressant drugs, cognitive therapy, financial and social help, and access to psychological and psychiatric expertise. Hormone therapy may help and it is often worth a trial after a diagnosis has been made. Probably the chief effect of oestrogen is in reducing vasomotor episodes and improving the sleep pattern. Women who sleep well can often show a considerable improvement in mood and their ability to cope with life. The Beck Inventory can be found in Appendix II.

General Health Questionnaire

The General Health Questionnaire was devised by Goldberg[2] to identify people in the community who were suffering from neurotic (non-psychotic) illness. The title is deliberately misleading in that there is no indication from the title that this is the purpose of the questionnaire, so that those who have a negative view of a diagnosis of psychiatric illness may not be deterred from answering the questions.

There are 140 items in the long form, 60 in the short and 12, 20 and 30 forms have been devised which contain the 'best items'. The 30-item questionnaire is overleaf and is self-administered.

Have you recently:

☐ been able to concentrate on whatever you're doing?

☐ lost much sleep over worry?

☐ felt that you are playing a useful part in things?

☐ felt capable of making decisions about things?

☐ felt constantly under strain?

☐ felt that you couldn't overcome your difficulties?

☐ been able to enjoy your normal day-to-day activities?

☐ been able to face up to your problems?

☐ been feeling unhappy or depressed?

☐ been losing confidence in yourself?

☐ been thinking of yourself as a worthwhile person?

☐ been feeling reasonably happy, all things considered?

☐ been managing to keep yourself busy and occupied?

☐ been getting out of the house as much as usual?

☐ been satisfied on the whole you were doing things well?

☐ been satisfied with the way you've carried out your tasks?

☐ been taking things hard?

☐ found everything getting on top of you?

☐ been feeling nervous and strung up all the time?

☐ found at times you couldn't do anything because your nerves were too bad?

☐ been having restless disturbed nights?

☐ been managing as well as most people would in your shoes?

☐ been able to feel warmth and affection for those near to you?

☐ been finding it easy to get on with other people?

☐ spent much time chatting with people?

☐ been finding it a struggle all the time?

☐ been getting scared or panicky for no good reason?

☐ felt that life is entirely hopeless?

☐ been feeling hopeful about your own future?

☐ felt that life isn't worthwhile?

The patients were asked to tick the appropriate box and when the questionnaire was completed it was scored as below:

Question	Less than usual	No more than usual	More than usual	Much more than usual
	0	**0**	**1**	**1**

The scores were added.

When large samples of men and women are tested, the total scores of the 30-question General Health Questionnaire in a 'normal' white population are shown in *Table 7.2*.

Table 7.2   Mean scores for the General Health Questionnaire

Age	Mean	SD
35-44	4.15	5.27
45-54	4.38	6.06
55-64	3.06	4.44
65-74	4.27	5.49

It is hoped that these questionnaires will be useful to readers who are dealing with the assessment of menopausal patients. They have all been validated and are used extensively by psychologists and medical workers in this country and abroad.

A further questionnaire which deals with the problems of depression and bereavement can be found in Appendix I, and Chapter 5 discusses psychological illness and the many severe problems faced by women of menopausal age.

References

1. Hunter M. The Women's Health Questionnaire: A measure of mid-aged women's perceptions of their emotional and physical health. *Psych & Health* 1992; **7**: 45-54.

2. Goldberg DP. *The Detection of Psychiatric Illness Questionnaire*. Oxford: Oxford University Press, 1972.

3. *The Lancet* (Editorial) 1995; **346** (July 1): 1-2.

4. Daly E, Gray A, Barlow D *et al.* Measuring the impact of menopausal symptoms on quality of life. *Br Med J* 1993: **307**: 836-40.

5. Beck AT, Ward CH, Mendleson M. An inventory for measuring depression. *Arch Gen Psych.* 1961: **4**: 561-70.

CHAPTER **EIGHT**

Care of patients following hysterectomy

W hen you refer the patient and hysterectomy is under discussion, it should be possible to request that healthy ovaries should be left *in situ*[1].

One week post-operation

At this stage the patient is probably still in hospital or about to return home. If the ovaries have been removed in a premenopausal patient, the consultant may initiate hormone therapy by inserting an oestradiol/testosterone implant at the time of the operation. Accurate transfer of information from hospital to general practitioner is important, including the findings at operation, whether ovaries were conserved and any treatment already commenced.

Contraindications to HRT include:

Breast cancer	Even this is not absolute and some patients with breast cancer are being entered for a randomised, controlled trial of HRT ± tamoxifen under specialist care.
Recent active thrombophlebitis	Thrombo-embolism, if treated with anti-coagulants, is not necessarily a contra-indication to HRT but specialist advice should be sought.
Endometriosis	may recur on HRT. Specialist supervision should be offered.

Two to four weeks post-operation

Usually the patient is at home and will need sickness insurance notes, wound care from the district nurse and general practitioner, and some domestic help. Physiotherapy is often useful in the form of a single teaching session. Because of the weakening of muscle and ligaments in the pelvic floor she should not lift weights for three months but many women can return to part-time desk work before this date.

Sexual intercourse may be resumed at five to six weeks with a lubricant, such as KY Jelly, as the patient has lost uterine secretion and the vagina may be very dry. Even if full penetration is not achieved at this stage it is important to attempt to re-establish the former pattern of intercourse as soon as possible. Discharge or bleeding should be reported to the general practitioner who may arrange vaginal swab culture or diathermy of granulomatous tissue in the vault. HRT improves vaginal dryness and the patient who does not wish to take systemic oestrogen may be treated with local oestrogen cream, pessaries or vaginal silicone/oestrogen rings.

Counselling about HRT

After oophorectomy

Time needs to be given to a full and frank discussion of the pros and cons of HRT. If the ovaries have been removed before the menopause, rapid bone loss can ensue and the patient needs long-term HRT to prevent osteoporosis and fractures[2] and lower the increased risk of heart disease[1,3].

Long-term HRT increases the risk of breast cancer if used over nine years[4] and some authorities would state five years[5]. However, the removal of both ovaries is highly protective against breast cancer so that on balance the benefit/risk ratio is positive in castrated patients for a period of at least 10 years or until the age of 50.

There should then be a discussion of possible methods of delivery, e.g. implant for patients with depressed libido (oestradiol 50 mg, testosterone 50 mg)[6], oestrogen patches such as *Evorel, Estraderm, Menorest* and *Fematrix* for patients likely to be intolerant of oral oestrogen (gall-bladder problems, hypertension etc.). The dose should be tailored to the patient; younger women may need 100-200 µg daily delivery of transdermal oestradiol, whereas older women may only tolerate 25-37.5 µg daily. Later a 'top-up' using oestrogen gel may be added to ensure increased flexibility of dose, particularly in women who are being weaned off an implant. Oral preparations are highly effective and conjugated equine oestrogens have been the preparations most commonly used in observational studies showing cardio-protection from long-term HRT[3].

Conserved ovaries

If the ovaries, or one ovary, have been left *in situ* the decision on HRT is not usually so urgent. FSH estimation is the guide as to whether ovarian function is present (*see p. 9*). If the values for FSH and LH are premenopausal it is unnecessary to begin HRT at this stage, although the patient will probably need some information and counselling. Transient flushes are common post-operatively but true ovarian failure may not occur for some years. There is disagreement over the question of whether simple hysterectomy advances the onset of ovarian failure. A recent study from Denmark[7] which examined bone density in hips and spine in 69 hysterectomised patients found no reduction in these women compared with matched controls. However, British workers have concluded that hysterectomy may cause early ovarian failure and bone loss[8]. It is useful for general practitioners to supervise their hysterectomised patients, whose names can be obtained by computer diagnostic printouts or exclusion from cervical smear screening lists, by offering FSH estimation every two to three years so that the onset of menopause can be established. At this date it is usual to offer further information and prescription of HRT, unless there is a contraindication.

It is vital to inform the patient fully and involve her in making decisions about therapy, otherwise she may be too anxious to comply with the recommended treatment. On the whole hysterectomised patients go on taking the treatment and have the highest rate of compliance[9].

The first prescription is usually for three months, when the patient is seen and questioned about possible side-effects and whether she feels well. If she is happy on the preparation chosen it can then be transferred to a long-term repeat prescription computerised list and she is seen yearly according to the programme already outlined. If the patient is experiencing unpleasant side-effects there is a wide range of preparations from which to choose an alternative. She does not need progestogen supplements. It is important to examine the breasts at each yearly visit, and after five years' HRT, to discuss the optimum length of therapy.

References

1.   van der Schouw YT, van der Graaf Y, Steyerberg EW *et al.* Age at menopause as a risk factor for cardiovascular mortality. *Lancet* 1996: **347**: 714-8.

2.   Cauley JA, Seeley DG, Ensrud K *et al.* Estrogen replacement therapy and fractures in older women. *Ann Int Med* 1995; **122**: 9-16.

3. Stampfer MK, Colditz GA, Willett WC *et al.* Post-menopausal estrogen therapy and coronary heart disease: ten year follow-up from the Nurses' Health Study. *New Engl J Med* 1991; **325**: 756-762.

4. Bergkvist I, Adami H-O, Persson I *et al.* The risk of breast cancer after estrogen and estrogen-progestin replacement. *New Engl J Med* 1989; **321**: 293-7.

5. McPherson K. Breast cancer and hormonal supplements in post-menopausal women. *Br Med J* 1995; **311**: 699-700.

6. Eccleston GA. Management of the menopause with hormone implants. *J Brit Men Soc* 1996; **2**(1): 9-14.

7. Ravn P, Lind C, Nilas L. Lack of influence of simple premenopausal hysterectomy on bone mass and bone metabolism. *Am J Obs & Gynaecol* 1995; **172.3**: 891-5.

8. Watson NR, Studd JWW, Garnett T *et al.* Bone loss after hysterectomy with ovarian conservation. *Obs & Gynaecol* 1995; **86.1**: 72-77.

9. Coope J, Marsh J. Can we improve compliance with long-term HRT? *Maturitas* 1992; **15**: 151-8.

CHAPTER **NINE**

Case studies

Case studies

T his chapter contains a series of case studies which illustrate some of the problems of managing the menopause and prescribing HRT. There has been no attempt to 'tidy them up'.

The patients are all real people who have presented with real problems over the past year in our general practice in Cheshire. The names have been altered to preserve confidentiality, and all the women have given permission for their case histories to be used in this way for teaching purposes.

Management of the menopause illustrates the inter-relatedness and the complexity of some of the clinical problems which are encountered every day in general practice.

- **Case Study 1**   Jane S, *aged 54*

- **Case Study 2**   Jean N, *aged 52*

- **Case Study 3**   Miriam K, *aged 66*

- **Case Study 4**   Geraldine E, *aged 66*

- **Case Study 5**   Sandra M, *aged 59*

- **Case Study 6**   Jennifer, *aged 52*

- **Case Study 7**   Elizabeth M, *aged 51*

- **Case Study 8**   Sheila E, *aged 56*

- **Case Study 9**   Barbara, *aged 70*

- **Case Study 10**   Mary R, *aged 66*

Case study 1

Jane S, aged 54

I am a housewife with six children aged 10-19. In *1987* I developed thyroid deficiency and started treatment with thyroxine. In *1989* a prolapse was diagnosed and also an abnormal cervical smear; I broke my arm that winter. The periods became very heavy and I was anaemic so I was referred to a gynaecologist. He carried out a hysterectomy via the vagina so that he could also repair the prolapse. The ovaries were not removed.

In *1991* the urine was very frequent and it felt as if the bladder was not emptying; the specialist did a cystoscopy but I was no better. They carried out more studies using filming of the bladder and found the bladder was very small.

In *1992* I had cystoscopy and the urethra was cut, also sigmoidoscopy and barium enema for bleeding and bowel pain. There was no improvement.

In *1993* a further barium enema showed diverticulum and a pelvic scan showed I had a tiny vagina with a band across and adhesions round the vagina. This explains why we have not been able to have sex much since the hysterectomy.

In *1993* I was referred to another specialist who put me on HRT and offered self-catheterisation which I refused. Lately I have been feeling unwell and frequently tired.

1994 Doctor's note

The oestradiol level in 1993 was very low. Bladder capacity 414 ml (low). Encouraged to use HRT.

June 1994. Very depressed. Sexual function poor. T4 92, TSH 43.3 (usually <5.0: myxodematous level). Looks hypothyroid. Oestradiol level 92 pmol/l despite taking *Premarin* 1.25 mg. Obviously interaction is occurring between oestrogen-raised thyroxine-binding globulin and thyroxine. Consult laboratory. Increase thyroxine to 100 µg daily.

Change to *Estraderm* patches.

Case study 2

Jean N, aged 52

Last year *(1994)* I went to see the doctor because I was suffering from flushes. I was in the process of separating from my husband and was very anxious over this and over the possession of the house. My father had died at the age of 59 of lung cancer. My last period was in October 1994.

In *May 1995* I bled from the vagina and was referred to a gynaecologist. He carried out a hysteroscopy in August 1995 and this was normal.

September 1995. Now I am feeling very tired with a lot of flushes and I wake up a lot. My previous experience of HRT (three years ago) was unpleasant and my breasts were painful. I don't smoke and take plenty of exercise with the dogs so I am fairly healthy.

October 1995 Doctor's note

She has had a further post-menopausal bleed despite recent normal hysteroscopy in July/August. The bleeding was very painful. ?Endometriosis, although a first diagnosis is rare after the menopause. The specialist has recommended cyclic progestogen, but she would prefer a definite diagnosis to be made before starting treatment. There may be some pathology in ovary, uterus or bladder (recently a woman in our practice with carcinoma of the bladder presented with what she mistook for bleeding from the vagina).

I have referred her for vaginal ultrasound examination. It is too early for HRT. If the scan shows endometrial thickness ≥8 mm she will need a biopsy.

Case study 3

Miriam K, aged 66

I am a retired headteacher aged 66, a non-smoker, married and live an active life with visits to grandchildren, walking and regular swimming with my husband. Asthma was diagnosed at the age of 30 and I took corticosteroids frequently in high dosage, usually as prednisolone 5-40 mg daily. At the age of 50 I started regular daily inhaled and oral corticosteroids, but have now reduced treatment and am stabilised on prednisolone 5 mg daily and *Intal* inhalations. As I was aware of the risk of osteoporosis I took *Premarin* 0.625 mg following hysterectomy for fibroids at the age of 47. The ovaries were not removed.

Five years later, at the age of 52, I developed bleeding from the breast and exploration showed hyperplasia of the duct so I was advised to stop HRT. There were no further breast symptoms and the mammogram was negative and has remained normal.

Later, in view of the risk of corticosteroid osteoporosis, I started oestrogen patches but I was advised to stop these after 10 years total use of oestrogen because of the accumulated increased risk of breast cancer after 10-15 years use which occurred in some American studies. Densitometry at the age of 60 and again at 65 was at the lower limit of normal.

Doctor's comment

At present this patient does not take HRT. She is being investigated for possible angina and breathlessness on exertion. If the exercise ECG is positive she wishes to re-start oestrogen therapy as the cardioprotective effect probably outweighs the increased risk of cancer. There is no relevant family history. BP, which was raised, is now controlled on bendrofluazide.

This case demonstrates the way that the decision on whether to take HRT depends on the presence of risk factors, such as bleeding from the breast (breast cancer) or corticosteroid use, particularly if this is continued for many years at high dosage (fracture risk). There is no problem about stopping and starting oestrogen treatment on condition that the patient accepts the probability of rebound flushing when HRT is withdrawn. HRT 'works' at any age and our oldest HRT user in the practice decided to take it when her fifth fracture occurred at the age of 80.

The next case illustrates that other partners may take the initiative in prescribing oestrogen if they are aware of the possible benefits.

Case study 4

Geraldine E, aged 66

Dr John suggested I take HRT. There is a history of heart disease in my family and he thought it might help to protect my heart. I have had angina for a number of years and my cholesterol level was quite high. I have taken HRT for about 12 months and I honestly do feel much better. I do not get the chest pain like I did before and my cholesterol level is down. I really feel much younger than my 66 years.

Doctor's comment

There is a family history of angina. Her brother died in 1972 after a coronary bypass operation. She has suffered from angina since 1985, when she was obese with BMI >30 and BP was raised. Despite dietary advice her cholesterol remained high with the following readings:

1991	Cholesterol 9.1	
1992	Cholesterol 7.4	
1993	Cholesterol 8.3	
1994	Fasting lipids. Cholesterol 8.1	Weight 81 kg
	BP 160/92	Triglycerides 2.68
	HDL-chol. 1.4 (0.9-2.1)	LDL-chol. 5.5 (2.5-5.8)

Aug 1994: *Premarin* 0.625 mg plus *Micronor* 700 µg daily was prescribed.

1994	Fasting cholesterol 6.7	Triglycerides 1.83
	HDL - 1.2	LDL - 4.7
April 1995	BP 166/92	Fasting cholesterol 6.2
		LDL - 4.7
Oct 1995	Cholesterol 5.8	
	After 11 months' HRT	
	HDL - 1.1	LDL - 3.9

She is well on continuous *Premarin* and *Micronor*. There is no bleeding and she does not want to change prescription. The dose of norethisterone is lower than in *Kliofem* or *Micronor* HRT. There has been steady improvement in the lipid pattern and also in her symptoms since she started HRT in August 1994.

Case study 5

Sandra M, aged 59

In *1974* I attended hospital for treatment for an erosion on my womb combined with heavy bleeding at menstrual time. The doctor decided that a hysterectomy was required because I also had something called chocolate cysts. They intended removing my womb but leaving me with both my ovaries. When I came round from the operation both my ovaries had been removed and I was told I would need to take hormone pills. Unfortunately, in 1974 there was not the same amount of information and help that there is available today. Doctors were very unsure of HRT and I commenced taking one *Premarin* a day, every day. Over the past 20 years I have tried various types of HRT including patches. At one stage I was swollen and painful so I returned to just patches. I have not had any adverse reaction to HRT over the 20 years. My only complaint is my urethra and too much protein in my water (whether this is just a side-effect of HRT I do not know). My next hurdle is when to come off HRT as I will be 60 years old next year. My biggest fear is breast cancer and I have regular checks when I collect my prescription every three months. I find this very helpful.

Doctor's comment

After hysterectomy and removal of both ovaries in 1974 she took *Premarin* 0.625 mg daily, sometimes with progestogen in addition. She was well apart from recurrent urinary tract infection which was investigated by mid-stream specimen of urine (MSSU) and cystoscopy in 1989, 1990 and 1994 - the last time urethral dilatation was carried out. Her mother had suffered from bladder cancer. In 1995 she complained of flushes on *Premarin* 0.625 mg and investigation showed oestradiol 121 pmol/l (low level). HRT was increased to *Premarin* 1.25 mg, but her breasts became very painful. Prescription was changed to *Premarin* 0.625 mg and *Evorel* patch 25. She is well on this but still has frequency, discomfort and smelly urine. MSSU: 100 leucocytes, no growth. A prescription of *Estring* has been given to prevent recurrent urinary symptoms, in addition to other HRT. There is evidence from controlled trials that local oestrogen improves genitourinary symptoms and prevents recurrent cystitis. She needs systemic HRT in full dosage in addition because both ovaries were removed at the age of 38.

Case study 6

Jennifer, aged 52 (a housewife with two teenage children)

I had always intended to cope with the menopause naturally - on a sort of 'mind over matter' basis. The decision to do otherwise came in July last year after some months of great stress.

My mother had died in May, after suffering from cancer of the colon for about 18 months. It was extremely distressing for her, and for my brother and me to have to watch. During this time my periods became very irregular, and they stopped after she died. I then started having hot flushes - they seemed to be occurring every 10 minutes or so, and I felt exhausted and depressed. My husband and I had arranged a holiday in the USA to visit his brother, and I felt it would be unfair to inflict my miserable self on them as I was - hence my decision to try HRT, if only to stop the hot flushes and mood swings.

HRT has certainly helped, although I am still experimenting with the brands. I put on weight with *Prempak-C* (or was I eating too much?). I do have to watch my blood pressure, and it was decided that I should try patches. The *Estracombi* seemed to give me irregular bleeding, so I am about to try *Estrapak* which delivers oestrogen by patch and progestogen by mouth. I have also tried *Tridestra*, which produces a bleed only every three months, but started getting a lot of dizzy spells (one of the side-effects warned about) so I decided to revert to the patches. I think I have been very fortunate that I have had so few side-effects, and am happy to continue for the time being.

I have had two children, both by Caesarean section, and suffered from post-natal depression after the first. My health has otherwise been reasonable, apart from a bad attack of labyrinthitis two years ago which, together with my mother's illness, put an end to my employment (I had been 13 years with the Citizens' Advice Bureau). I do need to keep busy, both mentally and physically, as I tend otherwise towards extreme lethargy. It follows that I do find it difficult to relax. I have the usual aches and pains to be expected at my age (52) but I swim regularly, walk a lot, and eat healthily, in an attempt to keep as fit as I can for as long as I can. I resist taking medication but do take vitamin supplements. My main fear is of developing cancer of the colon.

Doctor's comments

She had benign breast lumps and negative mammogram in 1984. When she took *Prempak-C* 0.625 mg in 1994 BP rose from 160/90 to 174/94 mmHg.

1995 - Estracombi. Well - BP 160/90 mmHg and remains at this level.

September 1995. Requested alteration of *Estrapak* or *Estracombi* schedules as she was going on holiday abroad for three months. Advised to use *Tridestra* which is safe and approved for this purpose of 3/12 bleeds. The dizzy spells which she experienced previously may be been connected with her attack of labyrinthitis and there is no evidence that they were associated with her use of *Tridestra*. It will be interesting to see if dizziness recurs on treatment.

Case study 7

Elizabeth M, aged 51

I usually enjoy very good health and have had no major problems. When I was 48 I was invited by my GP to attend a 'Well Woman's Clinic'. This was very instructive as it included not only a physical examination, but also advice about diet and the possible future use of HRT, its advantages and disadvantages. As a result, I read some magazine articles and listened to various radio programmes on the subject of HRT and decided that the positives, i.e. protection against osteoporosis, far outweighed the negatives.

Just after my 50th birthday I began to experience several mild hot flushes every day. My GP told me I was an ideal candidate for a new trial of HRT which the practice was involved in setting up. I was given several hundred pounds worth of free medical treatment including a mammogram and a vaginal ultrasound. My GP examined me thoroughly internally and externally, took my blood pressure, and blood and urine sample, and measured my height and weight. The tests proved satisfactory, the blood test showed I was menopausal, but a speck of blood was found in my urine. Further on-the-spot urine tests gave the same reading and a sample was sent to the laboratory. This final test proved to be satisfactory, but because of the time lapse it was necessary to take another blood sample. During this time the hot flushes had completely stopped and when the result of the second blood test came back it showed that I was not menopausal at all.

I was, therefore, unable to take part in the new HRT trial, but decided to accept HRT treatment as I feel the protection it provides against osteoporosis is invaluable.

I have now been taking HRT for three months and I cannot say that it has made a great deal of difference to my life. I do not feel 10 years younger, but neither have I experienced any unpleasant side-effects. During the first course I did experience a bad headache and very heavy bleeding, but this usually occurred during periods when I was a younger woman. Obviously my body will need time to adjust to HRT but I have every confidence that it is the correct way forward.

Doctor's comments

This patient consulted with typical menopausal symptoms and FSH was >100 iu/l, LH 12.0 iu/l, oestradiol 30 pmol/l. She was entered for a trial of a new form of combined oestrogen patch and screening involved mammography and vaginal ultrasound scan. The endometrium was <4 mm double thickness, ultrasound of the kidneys showed small cysts of the kidney of no real clinical significance, which probably accounted for microscopic haematuria found on urinalysis.

Repeat blood tests after six months showed FSH 16 iu/l, LH 3.0 iu/l, oestradiol 410 pmol/l (premenopausal level).

This patient still complained of flushes, but they were mild. She requested HRT and is now taking *Prempak*-C 0.625 mg.

This is an example of how 'menopausal' patients can regress to premenopausal state. We checked her method of contraception; her husband had had a vasectomy.

182

Case study 8

Sheila E, aged 56
a pleasant intelligent retired teacher,
married to an engineer;
her father died of a stroke

Sometime in my early 40s, I started to have frequent panic attacks, mood swings and lack of confidence in my abilities, resulting in hysterical bouts of crying and refusal to answer the doorbell and the telephone. I would run upstairs to hide should visitors call, rather than face them on my own. I would not go shopping locally in case I met someone I knew and was forced to talk to them, in fact I was always happier shopping in places where I was not known.

Initially, I was diagnosed as suffering from severe depression and prescribed antidepressants. The weeping bouts became more frequent and other symptoms continued. My husband tells me that my mood swings became worse and I could switch from being cheerful to being very unpleasant in a very short time but that the return to my more normal self took quite a long time. He describes it as like a chemical switch. I have no recollection of this aspect at all, which is just as well because he says that although the changes always took him by surprise and that most of the time he could cope because he knew I was not to blame, he admits that he sometimes made matters worse by retaliating. The whole thing eventually became so bad that on many occasions I could not cope with the thought of doing my job as a teacher and was very fortunate in having an extremely understanding and patient headmaster.

We made an appointment to see you and, as they say, "the rest is history". You interviewed us and then prescribed HRT. The pills that I had initially were on clinical trial and the improvement in my condition was virtually instantaneous. I returned to my normal gregarious self, my self-confidence returned and I felt I could face anyone and anything. My husband says that my mood swings disappeared completely at that stage but they did return, although to a very much lesser degree, when I was obliged to change to a different kind of pill.

Doctor's comments

In 1984 Sheila attended the well-woman clinic and asked for help with headaches, PMS and phobic anxiety. She was 45 years old and her periods were regular. She requested HRT and *Cyclo-Progynova* 2 mg was prescribed.

After a year, aged 46, she requested a higher dose because of flushes. BP was 160/110. *Prempak-C* 1.25 mg was prescribed and she felt very well, with regular bleeds. All subsequent BP readings were normal.

In 1993 she was 54, BP rose to 180/90. Monitoring showed mean level 132/71.

In 1994 her weight had risen to 10st and BP was 184/92. Bendrofluazide 2.5 mg daily was prescribed and the dose of oestrogen was reduced to *Prempak-C* 0.625 mg. Later that year she had a stroke with hemiplegia and is still hardly able to walk. Doppler investigation identified a carotid stenosis which was treated surgically. She is taking part in a rehabilitation programme and the surgeon has requested that she re-start HRT because of the beneficial effect of oestrogen on the arterial system. She has difficulty in reaching the toilet and undressing. So *Kliofem* (continuous oestrogen/progestogen) has been prescribed in order to avoid the inconvenience of 'periods'. At 56 she is assumed to be post-menopausal. Low-dose aspirin is also given and the blood pressure is checked frequently. There is no evidence that her stroke was associated with taking HRT. Epidemiological evidence suggests that oestrogen users are less likely to suffer a stroke, and that the use of oestrogen causes vasodilatation and protects the arteries.

Case study 9

Barbara, aged 70

I retired from work about 10 years ago and spend my time cooking for my husband and grandchildren and travelling the world to visit them. We have a son in Canada, married with a baby, and another son in Northumberland with four children. Our two daughters live close by. For about two years I have been developing low back pain which came and went. Last summer I was coming back from Canada and tried to lift my suitcase off the carousel at the airport. There was a sharp pain in my back and this did not improve over four weeks although I have had two treatments from the physiotherapist.

Doctor's comments

Barbara is a retired accountant aged 70. She is married and travels a great deal to see her grandchildren who live abroad. She was referred by the physiotherapist because of persistent low back pain which had continued for four months and had not responded to treatment.

An X-ray of the spine disclosed seven spinal fractures. She gave a history of an acute attack of lumbar pain in the thoracic-lumbar region which started when she lifted a suitcase off a carousel. It is likely that this episode represented the most recent fracture and that others had occurred silently over some months or years.

She is being treated with etidronate, and bone density, which was reduced, is being monitored at two-yearly intervals.

She requested HRT in addition and oestrogen/progestogen was prescribed but after a month she suffered an attack of biliary colic. The ultrasound examination showed gallstones and she was advised to stop HRT. She is still taking etidronate with three-monthly supervision and will probably change to alendronate in the near future.

She is a non-smoker and the menopause at 50 was not particularly early. The only possible contributing factor to her condition may be her dislike of sunlight and habit of staying indoors during summer. Since the diagnosis of spinal osteoporosis was confirmed she goes out more and her daughters help with the housework.

Case study 10

Mary R, aged 66

I am a happily married woman aged 66. I have two children and five grandchildren. When my mother was my age she suffered greatly with osteoporosis. That was 15 years ago and no one of my acquaintance had ever heard of osteoporosis and we had to explain it to everyone. She had other problems too, she needed a gall bladder operation and she was nearly blind with cataracts, but nothing could be done because of the fragility of her bones. She suffered so much that towards the end of her life I could not give her a hug and only the lightest of kisses as she was in such pain.

I finished my periods at 53, and 'put up' with the menopause for six years, then at 60 I had had enough of the hot flushes, sleeplessness and the dragging down feeling of getting older. So I went to talk it over with Dr Jean. She explained fully to me about the menopause and osteoporosis, and arranged X-rays and a scan for me, and advised HRT which I was most anxious to try. What a difference it has made to my life! Firstly, it has decreased my great fear of extreme osteoporosis that my dear mother suffered. Secondly, I feel younger and look much better. I am alert enough to carry on being a church organist frequently called upon to play in other churches as well as my own. I teach the keyboard and I create and sell crafts - handmade greetings cards, salt dough figures and novelties, I knit and sew for my grandchildren and take an active part in church affairs. The most important thing to me is that I feel a joy in living my life and speaking to my friends of all the benefits of HRT.

Doctor's comments

Mary contacted us because her mother suffered from severe osteoporosis before her death about 10 years previously. Her mother had a number of spinal fractures and the condition was so severe that on one occasion she reached down a jar from a shelf and felt a sharp pain due to another fracture.

Mary considered HRT at the age of 47 when she was still premenopausal and we suggested sequential oestrogen/progestogen, but she only decided

---

to take it at the age of 60. She also suffers from asthma and takes inhaled corticosteroids (beclomethasone 1 mg daily) and occasional prednisolone. When bone density measurements became available to the practice recently she was tested and found to have spinal bone density of 2.3 SD below the mean for her age. She had been taking HRT for six years. Because of the adverse family history she has received an additional prescription for biphosphonates - *Didronel PMO*, which is to be taken concurrently with HRT. We intend to monitor bone density every two to three years and keep the corticosteroid treatment at as low a level as possible. As more preparations become available the biphosphonate may be changed for alendronate or other similar drug. As she is now post-menopausal we can offer HRT as continuous oestrogen and progestogen which does not cause 'periods' (*Kliofem*). Mary does not smoke and eats a normal diet with added calcium. She exercises out of doors and is very active with her grandchildren who live locally. She was already aware of the risk of osteoporosis because of the family history and our chief difficulty has been in obtaining bone density measurement to confirm the diagnosis. It is presumed that treatment with biphosphonate will offer additional protection to that provided by HRT and further research is awaited. She has not suffered a fracture and her health is enormously better than that of her mother at the same age.

These case notes have been chosen to show some of the problems which face doctors who are managing menopausal patients and prescribing hormone therapy. However, most of our patients do not have difficulty in deciding about HRT and our practice of 10,000 patients has over 300 HRT users who attend for routine checks and are reasonably well and happy about their treatment. All middle-aged women are encouraged to attend for education and advice, but individuals are left to make their own decision as to whether to take hormones after adequate information and screening from the doctor and nurse.

EPILOGUE

Many women sail through the menopause without symptoms and feel that they do not want to medicalise their lives by taking drugs. Others are badly affected by lack of sleep and the social hazard of hot flushes, and are grateful for therapy.

The duration of the treatment to prevent heart disease or fractures is the subject of debate. Women who have their ovaries irradiated or removed before the menopause should take HRT until at least the age of 50 unless there is an over-riding contraindication, such as untreated breast cancer. Oestrogen can be considered for adequately treated early stage breast cancer patients but they should be entered into an appropriate trial. It was formerly believed that eight years of HRT given within three years of menopause would give lifelong reduction of fracture risk. It now seems that much longer treatment may be required to provide maximal protection against heart disease and osteoporosis[1].

Preventive health care for a geriatric population was discussed recently in the *Lancet* and it is appropriate to end with a quotation from the article by Patterson and Chambers[2], which lists HRT as offering secondary prevention with fair evidence of benefit.

'Oestrogen replacement

Differential rates of morbidity and mortality from cardiovascular disease in men and women converge after the menopause. Meta-analysis of prospective cohort studies of cardiovascular mortality conclude that the relative risk of cardiovascular death or morbidity is reduced in women who have used oestrogen replacement. Osteoporosis and its common complications (fractures of the distal radius, vertebrae and hip) are common in menopausal women. Evidence from randomised controlled trials shows that hormonal replacement prevents bone loss and may reduce the risk of osteoporotic fractures in perimenopausal women up to 10 years post-menopause. Balanced against these benefits is a possible small increase in the risk of breast cancer and an increased risk of carcinoma of the body of the uterus in those given unopposed oestrogens. Counselling concerning individual risks and benefits of hormone replacement is recommended for all post-menopausal women.'

References

1. Drife JO. Benefits and risks of hormone replacement therapy - an update. *Ad Drug Bull* 1994; **166**: 627-30.

2. Patterson C, Chambers LW. Preventive health care. *Lancet* 1995; **345**: 1611-5.

APPENDIX I

Quality of Life Questionnnaire

Quality of Life Questionnaire

We would like you to begin by listening carefully to two short statements: the first describes what it might be like to experience mild menopausal symptoms, the second what it might be like to experience severe menopausal symptoms.

Mild menopausal symptoms may take **one** of the following forms:

- You will have occasional hot flushes once or twice a day and night sweats which will wake you up occasionally. These may last for between six months and five or even 10 years.

or
- Your concentration and confidence will be poorer than a few years ago, you will cope less well with your job or other work, and you will feel tired some of the time. This may last for between six months and five or even 10 years.

or
- You will notice that your vagina is rather dry and that this makes sex a little painful. This could continue for a long time, perhaps the rest of your life. You will be less interested in sex than you used to be.

Severe menopausal symptoms may take **one or all** of the following forms:

- You will have severe menopausal flushing once or twice every hour with night sweats every night, causing you to lose sleep and often causing you to change your nightdress.

- You will feel very severe tiredness accompanied by a lack of concentration and confidence so great that you are failing to cope not only with your work, but also with your home life, with effects on the relationships in your family.

- You will experience complete lack of interest in sex which is only partly because of vaginal dryness. Your lack of interest is so great that you feel even if the vagina was not dry you would not positively choose to have sex. This problem will be seriously affecting your marriage.

Rating scale measurement technique

The first question we would like to ask you is:

"How would you rate your overall quality of life if you were experiencing these symptoms: the scale runs from 0 to 10, 10 being equivalent to normal health and 0 being dead."

Quality of Life scale

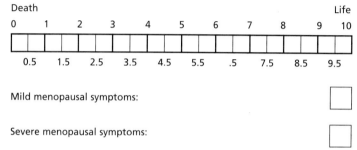

Mild menopausal symptoms:

Severe menopausal symptoms:

Trade-off measurement technique

Now we would like you to imagine that you are able to make a choice between having these symptoms for a certain period of time, and being in full health for a shorter period of time: in other words, you can make a trade-off between the length of life and the quality of life.

We would now like to ask you a number of hypothetical questions about this trade-off.

First, listen again to the description of mild menopausal symptoms.

Mild menopausal symptoms may take **one** of the following forms:

- • You will have occasional hot flushes once or twice a day and night sweats which will wake you up occasionally. These may last for between six months and five or even 10 years.

or
- • Your concentration and confidence will be poorer than a few years ago, you will cope less well with your job or other work, and you will feel tired some of the time. This may last for between six months and five or even 10 years.

159

or
- You will notice that your vagina is rather dry and that this makes sex a little painful. This could continue for a long time, perhaps the rest of your life. You will be less interested in sex than you used to be.

Now, what would you choose between five years of mild menopausal symptoms and five years of normal health?

What would you choose between five years of mild menopausal symptoms and 4.5 years of normal health?

What would you choose between five years of mild menopausal symptoms and 4 years of normal health?

What would you choose between five years of mild menopausal symptoms and 3.5 years of normal health?

- Continue until a point is reached when the interviewee is indifferent between the choices available. Interviewer will also use months as point of indifference is approached.

Mild symptoms: indifference point (years/months):

Next, listen again to the description of severe menopausal symptoms.

Severe menopausal symptoms may take **one or all** of the following forms:

- You will have severe menopausal flushing once or twice every hour with night sweats every night, causing you to lose sleep and often causing you to change your nightdress.

- You will feel very severe tiredness accompanied by a lack of concentration and confidence so great that you are failing to cope not only with your work, but also with your home life, with effects on the relationships in your family.

- You will experience complete lack of interest in sex which is only partly because of vaginal dryness. Your lack of interest is so great that you feel even if the vagina was not dry you would not positively choose to have sex. This problem will be seriously affecting your marriage.

Now, what would you choose between five years of severe menopausal symptoms and five years of normal health?

What would you choose between five years of severe menopausal symptoms and 4.5 years of normal health?

What would you choose between five years of severe menopausal symptoms and 4 years of normal health?

What would you choose between five years of severe menopausal symptoms and 3.5 years of normal health?

- Continue until a point is reached when the interviewee is indifferent between the choices available. Interviewer will also use months as point of indifference is approached.

Severe symptoms: indifference point (years/months):

Time trade-off method

Years of menopausal symptoms   Years of normal health

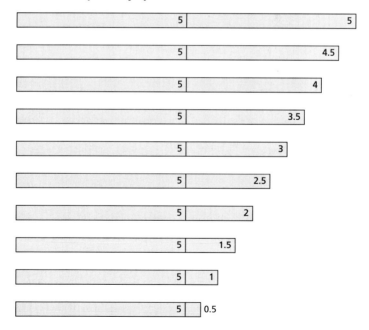

Would you consider yourself as someone who has suffered from:

Severe menopausal symptoms?   No = 0, Yes = 1   ☐

If no above:
Mild menopausal symptoms?   No = 0, Yes = 1   ☐

If yes to one of above:
Do you think that the description of (severe/mild) menopausal symptoms given earlier in this exercise accurately describes your own experience?

No = 0, Yes = 1   ☐

If no to above:
Do you think that the description overstated or understated the symptoms you have experienced?

Understand = 0, Overstated = 1   ☐

If yes to having experienced mild or severe symptoms:
Have you received HRT as a treatment for your menopausal symptoms?

No = 0, Yes = 1   ☐

If yes to above:
How would you rate your overall quality of life before and after you began HRT, on a scale running from 0 to 10, with 10 being equivalent to normal health and 0 being dead.

Before HRT   ☐

After HRT   ☐

There are no more questions; would you like to make any comments relating to this exercise or to HRT?

Daly E, Gray A, Barlow D *et al*. Measuring the impact of menopausal symptoms on quality of life. *Br Med J* 1993: **317**: 836-40.

Reproduced with the permission of the authors.

APPENDIX II

Beck Depression Inventory

Depression inventory

A   0. I do not feel sad.
1. I feel blue or sad.
2. I am blue or sad all the time and I can't snap out of it.
2. I am so sad or unhappy that it is very painful.
3. I am so sad or unhappy that I can't stand it.

B   0. I am not particularly pessimistic or discouraged about the future.
1. I feel discouraged about the future.
2. I feel I have nothing to look forward to.
2. I feel that I won't ever get over my troubles.
3. I feel that the future is hopeless and that things cannot improve.

C   0. I do not feel like a failure.
1. I feel I have failed more than the average person.
2. I feel I have accomplished very little that is worthwhile
or that means anything.
2. As I look back on my life all I can see is a lot of failures.
3. I feel I am a complete failure as a person (parent, husband/wife).

D   0. I am not particularly dissatisfied.
1. I feel bored most of the time.
1. I don't enjoy things the way I used to.
2. I don't get satisfaction out of anything any more.
3. I am dissatisfied with everything.

E   0. I don't feel particularly guilty.
1. I feel bad or unworthy a good part of the time.
2. I feel quite guilty.
2. I feel bad or unworthy practically all the time now.
3. I feel as though I am very bad or worthless.

F   0. I don't feel I am being punished.
1. I have a feeling that something bad may happen to me.
2. I feel I am being punished or will be punished.
3. I feel I deserve to be punished.
3. I want to be punished.

G   0. I don't feel disappointed in myself.
1. I am disappointed in myself.
1. I don't like myself.
2. I am disgusted with myself.
3. I hate myself.

H   0. I don't feel I am any worse than anybody else.
       1. I am very critical of myself for my weaknesses or mistakes.
       2. I blame myself for everything that goes wrong.
       2. I feel I have many bad faults.

I   0. I don't have any thoughts of harming myself.
       1. I have thoughts of harming myself but I would not carry them out.
       2. I feel I would be better off dead.
       2. I have definite plans about committing suicide.
       2. I feel my family would be better off if I were dead.
       3. I would kill myself if I could.

J   0. I don't cry any more than usual.
       1. I cry more now than I used to.
       2. I cry all the time now. I can't stop it.
       3. I used to be able to cry but now I can't cry at all even though I want to.

K   0. I am no more irritated now than I ever was.
       1. I get annoyed or irritated more easily than I used to.
       2. I feel irritated all the time.
       3. I don't get irritated at all at the things that used to irritate me.

L   0. I have not lost interest in other people.
       1. I am less interested in other people now than I used to be.
       2. I have lost most of my interest in other people
          and have little feeling for them.
       3. I have lost all my interest in other people
          and don't care about them at all.

M   0. I make decisions about as well as ever.
       1. I am less sure of myself now and try to put off making decisions.
       3. I can't make any decisions at all any more.

N   0. I don't feel I look any worse than I used to.
       1. I am worried that I am looking old or unattractive.
       2. I feel that there are permanent changes in my appearance
          and they make me look unattractive.
       3. I feel that I am ugly or repulsive looking.

O   0. I can work about as well as before.
       1. It takes extra effort to get started at doing something.
       1. I don't work as well as I used to.
       2. I have to push myself very hard to do anything.
       3. I can't do any work at all.

P   0. I can sleep as well as usual.
1. I wake up more tired in the morning than I used to.
2. I wake up 1-2 hours earlier than usual
and find it hard to get back to sleep.
3. I wake up early every day and can't get more than five hours sleep.

Q   0. I don't get any more tired than usual.
1. I get tired more easily than I used to.
2. I get tired from doing anything.
2. I get too tired to do anything.

R   0. My appetite is no worse than usual.
1. My appetite is not as good as it used to be.
2. My appetite is much worse now.
3. I have no appetite at all any more.

S   0. I haven't lost much weight, if any, lately.
1. I have lost more than five pounds.
2. I have lost more than 10 pounds.
3. I have lost more than 15 pounds.

T   0. I am no more concerned about my health than usual.
1. I am concerned about aches and pains or upset stomach or
constipation or other unpleasant feelings in my body.
2. I am so concerned with how I feel or what I feel that it's hard
to think of much else.
3. I am completely absorbed in what I feel.

U   0. I have not noticed any recent change in my interest in sex.
1. I am less interested in sex than I used to be.
2. I am much less interested in sex now.
3. I have lost interest in sex completely.

The score to be allotted to each answer appears alongside. When the scores
are added together the total score gives an indication of the presence or
absence and depth of depressive illness:

Table A2.1   Clinical rating of depth of depression corresponding to inventory score

	NONE	MILD	MODERATE	SEVERE
Mean score	10.9	18.7	25.4	30.0
(SD)	(8.1)	(10.2)	(9.6)	(10.6)

Mean scores are shown in Table A2.1, but the wide standard deviations should encourage physicians to assess patients as ill at slightly lower levels of total score. I have made a practice of referring patients for psychiatric help at total scores over 20, particularly if there is evidence of suicidal intent.

Beck AT, Ward CH, Mendleson M. An inventory for measuring depression. *Arch Gen Psych* 1961; **4**: 561-70.

Further reading

Further reading

For GPs

Khaw KT (ed). HRT. *British Medical Bulletin* **48** (2). British Medical Council. Edinburgh: Churchill Livingstone, 1992.

Assessment of fracture risk and its application to screening for post-menopausal osteoporosis. Report of WHO Study Group. WHO: Geneva, 1994.

McPherson A (ed). *Women's problems in general practice, third edition*. Oxford: Oxford University Press, 1993. (4th edition in press)

Coope J. *Hormone replacement therapy*. London: Royal College of General Practitioners, 1993.

Berg G, Hammar M (eds). *The modern management of the menopause. A perspective for the 21st Century*. Carnforth: Parthenon Publishing Group, 1994.

For patients

Hunter M, Coope J. *Time of her life*. London: Penguin Books, 1995.

Coope J. *The menopause: coping with the change*. London: Optima.

Graham-Smith E. *Exercises that work for you*. Wilmslow: Sigma Press, 1995.

INDEX

loss
  combined oral
  contraception 33
  HRT 45-6
  hysterectomy and 131, 132
  norethisterone 66
  low bone mass, definition 42
  normal, definition 42
  see also Osteoporosis
Bone mass
  loss after menopause 75
  low 42
  peak 43, 75
Bone mineral content (BMC) 42
Bone mineral density (BMD) 42
Boston Collaborative Group
Surveillance Program 51-2
Breast cancer
  anxiety about 59
  family history
    and HRT 96
    meta-analyses 55-6
    screening 59
  mortality, and HRT 55, 59
  Nurses' Health Study 54-5
  oestrogen and/or tamoxifen 57
  patients with 57
    and HRT 60, 95, 130
    survival 57
    and tamoxifen 57
  quality of life 122
  risk of
    and HRT 54-7, 55, 59, 99, 131, 139
    lifetime 54
  Royal Marsden Hospital's advice
  to GPs 59-60
Breast cysts 96

Breast disorders, benign 56, 96
Breast enlargement 101
Breast surgeons 93
Breathing, deep, and hot flushes 25
British Menopause Society 98
British Menopause Society,
Journal of 56, 88

C
Calcium 43
  antenatal 75
  dietary 43, 44, 105
  supplements 43
Cardiac valve disease 95
Cardiologists 93
Cardioprotection 52, 139, 141
  see also Ischaemic heart disease
Case studies 136-51
  cardioprotective effect 139, 141
  depression 147-8
  effect on thyroid
  hormones 137
  HRT and stroke 147-8
  post-menopausal bleeding 138
  prevention of
  osteoporosis 150-1
  regression to
  premenopausal state 145-6
  side-effects 142, 143-4
  spinal osteoporosis 149
Centre for Epidemiological Studies
Depression Scale (CES-D) 86
Cervical smears, abnormal 96
Cervical stenosis 35
Cholesterol 141
  Kliofem 70
CHUSE advice 43